Adaptive

and

Flexible Clinical Trials

Adaptive

and

Flexible Clinical Trials

Richard Chin

Institute for OneWorld Health
UCSF School of Medicine
San Francisco, California, USA

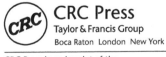

CRC Press
Taylor & Francis Group
Boca Raton London New York

CRC Press is an imprint of the
Taylor & Francis Group, an **informa** business

A CHAPMAN & HALL BOOK

CRC Press
Taylor & Francis Group
6000 Broken Sound Parkway NW, Suite 300
Boca Raton, FL 33487-2742

First issued in paperback 2019

© 2012 by Taylor & Francis Group, LLC
CRC Press is an imprint of Taylor & Francis Group, an Informa business

No claim to original U.S. Government works

ISBN-13: 978-1-4398-3832-7 (hbk)
ISBN-13: 978-0-367-38247-6 (pbk)

Visit the Taylor & Francis Web site at
http://www.taylorandfrancis.com

and the CRC Press Web site at
http://www.crcpress.com

This book is dedicated to my loving wife

for her unwavering support.

Contents

Introduction xi
About the Author xiii

1. Background 1
    1.1   Introduction 1
    1.2   Definition and History of Traditional Clinical Trials 2
    1.3   Definition of Adaptive Clinical Trial 5
    1.4   Precursors to Modern Adaptive Clinical Trials 10
    1.5   New Enabling Technologies and Other Requirements for
           Adaptive Trials 13
    1.6   Rationale for Adaptive Clinical Trials 14
    1.7   Learn and Confirm 16
    1.8   Classification and Terminology of Adaptive Clinical Studies 20
    1.9   Non-Adaptive Study Designs 21
    1.10 Limitations of Adaptive Clinical Trials 21
    1.11 Performance Criteria for Well-Designed Clinical Trials 22
    1.12 Evolving Regulatory Environment for Adaptive Clinical
           Trials 27
    1.13 Regulatory Guidance from the FDA 30
    References 36

2. Conventional Statistics 37
    2.1   Basic Statistics 37
    2.2   Statistical Schools 37
    2.3   Frequentist Method 38
    2.4   Bayesian Method 40
    2.5   Likelihood Method 40
    2.6   Other Schools 41
    2.7   Descriptive Statistics 41
    2.8   Inferential Statistics 41
    2.9   Comparative Statistics 43
    2.10 Hypothesis Testing 44
    2.11 Null Hypothesis and Standard of Proof in Clinical Trials 44
    2.12 Example of Inference and Hypothesis Testing 45
    2.13 Statistical Tests and Choice of Statistical Test 47
    2.14 Examples of Statistical Tests 48
    2.15 Fundamental Statistical Assumptions 50
           2.15.1 Background 50
           2.15.2 Parametric Assumption 52

2.15.3 Continuity and Linearity Assumptions 53
2.15.4 Constant Hazard Ratio Assumptions 53
2.15.5 Independent and Random Sampling 53
2.15.6 Independence of Events 54

3. Statistics Used in Adaptive Clinical Trials 55
   3.1   Introduction 55
   3.2   Preserving the Alpha 55
   3.3   What Is Alpha? 56
   3.4   Misconception about *p* Values 58
   3.5   Splitting the Alpha 59
   3.6   Methodologies for Allocating Alpha 60
          3.6.1 Bonferroni Correction 60
          3.6.2 Holm Correction 61
          3.6.3 Other Methods 61
   3.7   Evolution of Adaptive Analytic Methods: Interim Analysis 62
   3.8   Adaptive Methods 65
   3.9   Limitations of Adaptive Statistical Techniques 69
   3.10   Bayesian Approach 71
   3.11   Simulations and Modeling 72
   3.12   The FDA's Stance on Adaptive Techniques 73
   References 93

4. Specific Requirements for Adaptive Trials 95
   4.1   Requirements for Endpoints in Adaptive Studies 95
   4.2   Surrogates and Biomarkers 97
   4.3   Practical Requirements 99

5. Adaptive Randomization and Allocation 101
   5.1   Traditional Fixed Allocation 101
   5.2   Simple Randomization 102
   5.3   Restricted and Blocked Randomization 102
   5.4   Stratified, Nested, and Similar Randomization 103
   5.5   Balancing (Covariate) Adaptive Randomization 104
   5.6   Response (Outcome) Adaptive Randomization 105
   5.7   Combination and Multimodal Randomization 106
   5.8   Bayesian Randomization 107
   5.9   Adaptation of Inclusion and Exclusion Criteria Based on
          Blinded Data 107
   5.10   Patient Enrichment Adaptations 108

6. Sample Size Reestimation 111
   6.1   Background 111
   6.2   Sample Size Reestimation Based on Blinded Data 112

6.3 Sample Size Reestimation Based on Unblinded Data 113
6.4 Adjustment in Follow-Up Time 114
6.5 Internal Pilot Studies 114
6.6 Additional Rules 115
References 115

7. **Traditional Dosing** 117
7.1 Introduction 117
7.2 Definitions and Objectives of Dose Selection 118
7.3 Issues 119
7.4 Pharmacokinetics 120
7.5 Factors Affecting Pharmacokinetics 122
7.6 Dose–Response Curves 122
7.7 Types of Dosing 123
     7.7.1 Flat Doses 123
     7.7.2 Dosing Based on a Baseline Characteristic 124
     7.7.3 Titrated Dosing 124
7.8 Traditional Dose-Escalation and Dose-Ranging Studies 124

8. **Adaptive Dosing** 129
8.1 Adaptive Dose Finding 129
8.2 Phase I Studies 131
8.3 3 + 3 and Related Designs 132
8.4 Continual Reassessment Method 134
8.5 Dose Escalation with Overdose Control 137
8.6 Stochastic Approximation Methods 138
8.7 Summary of Single-Parameter Models 138
8.8 Additional Models and Methods 139
8.9 Dose Adaptation in a Pivotal Study 140
8.10 Changes in Concomitant Medications and Procedures 141
References 141

9. **Interim Analysis and Adaptive Termination of Study and Study Arms** 143
9.1 Overview 143
9.2 Data and Safety Monitoring Boards 143
9.3 Stopping Rules 145
9.4 Individual Sequential Designs 145
9.5 Group Sequential Designs 146
References 147

10. **Adaptive Changes in Study Design and Decision Rules** 149
10.1 Overview 149
10.2 Changes to Follow-Up Period 149

10.3   Flexible Designs 149
10.4   Changing the Endpoints and Hypothesis 150
       10.4.1   Changes Based on Blinded Data 150
       10.4.2   Changes Based on Unblinded Data 150
10.5   Changes to Test Statistic or Analysis 151
       10.5.1   Changes Based on Blinded Data 151
       10.5.2   Changes Based on Unblinded Data 151
References 152

11. Seamless Designs and Adaptive Clinical Trial Conduct 155
11.1   Seamless Designs 155
11.2   Challenges in Adaptive Trials 156
11.3   Maintaining the Blind 156
11.4   Infrastructure and Operations 157
11.5   Adaptive Trial Protocols 159

12. Analysis and Interpretation of Results 163
12.1   General Issues in Interpretation of Clinical Trial Results 163
12.2   Interpretation of Adaptive Trial Results 169
12.3   Documentation of Trial Integrity 170
12.4   Statistics of Adaptive Trial Analysis 171
12.5   Summary 172
References 172

Index 173

Introduction

Adaptive clinical trials, sometimes also called flexible clinical trials, are clinical studies that offer the ability to change study parameters during the course of the study. These studies differ from traditional studies in that rather than sample size(s), patient populations, endpoints, and other parameters being fixed at the beginning of the study, adaptive clinical studies allow for changes in one or more of these factors during the course of the study. Importantly, these changes are performed in such a way that they do not jeopardize the statistical validity of the study results.

Although the roots of adaptive studies can be traced back to methods developed decades ago, only recently have they become practical and popular, for reasons that will be explored later in the book. Some early methodologies for adaptation that have been used for decades include adaptive randomization and interim analysis. Interim analysis in particular, typically performed for the purposes of insuring patient safety, set some of the key statistical foundations that have led to modern adaptive study designs.

Some types of clinical studies, especially Phase I studies and oncology studies, have utilized adaptive designs or semi-adaptive designs for decades as well. However, they sometimes used less than rigorous statistical techniques and generally were not robust to the degree that would make the studies appropriate or acceptable for hypothesis-testing studies. Rather, they were used in a semi-informal manner for exploratory studies, with non-adaptive designs being *de rigueur* even for oncology studies.

The adaptive clinical trial, in its modern form, however, is a relatively new phenomenon and is an active area of methodological innovation. It is also advancing and changing rapidly. Statistical innovations, regulatory innovations, and operational innovations are all in a state of flux. This textbook attempts to capture the state of art in each of these areas.

There are many advantages to adaptive and flexible clinical trials. Although not a panacea, and while there are still some significant questions and issues that need to be addressed regarding acceptability and appropriateness of adaptive clinical trials in different circumstances, flexible and adaptive designs offer the potential for a much more efficient, ethical, and productive approach to clinical development.

To date, most of the available textbooks on adaptive clinical trials have been written with the statistician in mind. This is likely because in order for adaptive clinical studies to be designed, conducted, and accepted, the statistical and theoretical underpinnings are necessary. Now that such underpinnings have been relatively well developed, there is a need for a textbook that can be readily understood and utilized by clinicians and others who are not statistical experts.

This book is designed for clinical trialists, medical directors, data mangers, clinical operations personnel, and other non-statisticians involved in the design, conduct, and analysis of adaptive clinical research. The purpose of the book is not to teach the practical statistical methods to enable the reader to perform the analysis or simulations for adaptive trials but rather to teach the principles of adaptive design so that the reader can select and design the appropriate adaptive clinical trial designs from a conceptual perspective. By necessity, statistical concepts are described and discussed, including statistical concepts underlying traditional clinical trials as well as adaptive designs. Without a sound understanding of the statistical basis of both types of trials, it is impossible to understand and utilize adaptive clinical trials. However, the focus of the book is not on the mathematical details of those concepts but rather on the application of those concepts.

About the Author

Dr. Richard Chin is an internist with extensive expertise in drug development. He has overseen more than forty-five Investigational New Drug (IND) Applications for new molecular entities and new indications, as well as ten New Drug Applications (NDAs)/Biologic License Applications (BLAs)/ registration filings. He is currently CEO of OneWorld Health, a nonprofit biopharmaceutical company that develops affordable drugs for the most impoverished patients in the developing world. Previously, Dr. Chin was CEO of Oxigene, senior vice president of Global Development at Elan, and head of clinical research for the Biotherapeutics Unit at Genentech. He was named by *Businessweek* in 2006 as one of the ninety-nine youngest CEOs of public companies in the United States.

Dr. Chin received a B.A. in biology, *magna cum laude*, from Harvard University and the equivalent of a J.D. with honors from Oxford University in England under a Rhodes Scholarship. Dr. Chin holds a medical degree from Harvard Medical School and is licensed to practice medicine in California. He is currently on faculty of UCSF and was previously on the adjunct faculty at Stanford, and has authored a major textbook on clinical trial medicine. He currently serves on the boards of directors of RXi Pharmaceuticals, an RNAi company developing novel treatments for human diseases, and of Genmedica Therapeutics, a leading biotech company in Spain developing innovative treatments for diabetes. Dr. Chin may be contacted at richardchin@clinicaltrialist.com.

1

Background

1.1 Introduction

One of the most exciting new developments in clinical trial medicine is the emergence of adaptive and flexible clinical trials. The recent maturation of tools necessary for adaptive clinical trials—in particular the development of real-time, Web-based, electronic data entry systems as well as recent advances in statistical methods—has made adaptive clinical trials practical and attractive. Previously, most studies used paper-based case report forms that require weeks or months of time between patient visits and availability of data. Now, modern electronic data capture technology can shorten that time to days or hours. The rapid turnaround between data generation and data availability means that the progress of study can be monitored in real time. This means that the data and the analysis of the data, including endpoints, patient characteristics, and other parameters necessary to make changes in the study can be made available in real time. Without timely availability of these parameters, adaptive clinical studies are not possible.

Also, with modern statistical techniques, it has now become possible to alter, on the fly, almost any parameter of a study, including sample sizes, doses, treatment arms, randomization ratios, inclusion criteria, visit schedules, null hypothesis, analysis, and so on. We should distinguish between alterations of such parameters in adaptive designs where statistical validity is preserved, and inappropriate alteration of those parameters in non-adaptive clinical studies where the changes are made on an ad hoc basis and jeopardize the interpretability and validity of the study.

In addition to development of electronic data capture and maturation of necessary statistical techniques, the other important impetus for the growth of adaptive and flexible clinical trials has been the cost and length of modern clinical trials. Over the last two decades, there have been rapid and unsustainable increases in the cost of clinical development. The costs have been increasing at 20% per year or more. Such rapid escalation of costs is encouraging sponsors to look for ways of decreasing cost and timelines for developing drugs. Because adaptive designs can substantially lower the size of studies, and in many cases can lead to timely termination of studies with low probability of success, more and more corporate sponsors are turning to such designs.

The field of adaptive and flexible clinical trials is nascent, but there is an enormous amount of interest in it from clinical researchers. There have been numerous recent studies that have incorporated adaptive designs. There have been multiple international conferences devoted to adaptive studies. There is also growing interest from regulators such as the U.S. Food and Drug Administration (FDA) and the European Medicines Agency (EMA), both of which have published recent guidelines on adaptive and flexible clinical trials. While the field is new, there is no doubt that many clinical trials are shifting, where appropriate, to the new model of adaptive clinical trials.

1.2 Definition and History of Traditional Clinical Trials

Before defining adaptive and flexible clinical trials, it is important to examine and to understand the traditional method of developing drugs. The anatomy and evolution of classical, or non-adaptive, clinical trial methodology was based on a set of constraints and needs. Understanding why classical clinical trial designs were fashioned in a certain way illuminates the ways where they can be improved and where they cannot.

Classically, clinical trials have been divided into three phases: Phase I, Phase II, and Phase III.

Phase I studies were designed to identify or elucidate the maximally tolerated dose, adverse effects, pharmacokinetics (PK) parameters and pharmacodynamic (PD) parameters. They were primarily intended to gingerly test the toxicity of the drug. They were usually performed in volunteers, although in some instances, such as with biologics or with antineoplastic agents, Phase I studies have often been performed in patients.

Phase II studies have been a lot more heterogeneous in form and substance than Phase I trials, but in general, they have been designed to define the appropriate dose, gather additional data on safety, and if possible, to establish proof of concept.

Phase III studies have been utilized to establish both safety and efficacy, to the extent this is possible in the context of a clinical trial setting.

The so-called Phase IV studies have been studies performed after approval, usually to gather additional safety data or to establish effectiveness in the clinical practice setting.

There are some additional variations on the phases, such as Phase 0 studies, which are microdose studies performed with very small doses of the drug, and Phase IIIb studies, designed to add indications, but the Phase I/II/III model has been the standard approach to drug development for several decades.

The three phases evolved out of specific needs, and were developed on the basis of available technologies at the time when clinical trials in its modern form arose.

The Phase I studies arose because of a need to gingerly test potentially toxic drugs for the first time in people. Even today, Phase I is the most dangerous phase for patients in clinical studies. No matter how thoroughly the drug has been tested in animals, it is impossible to insure that the drug will not be highly toxic to people. Because of the risks involved in first-in-man studies, namely death and injury, Phase I has to be conducted in a slow, gently escalating fashion with just a few patients. However, Phase I studies are not hypothesis testing, and have less severe statistical constraints. Because of the risk, the small size of the studies that have made real-time data analysis practicable, and because of fewer statistical constraints, Phase I studies have often been adaptive.

Phase II studies exist to minimize significant amounts of money and time invested in Phase III studies. This is favored by most sponsors who want to de-risk the program and refine the dose and endpoints to reduce the size of Phase III studies. Phase II studies do not necessarily have to be hypothesis testing, but often are designed as hypothesis testing studies, because that reduces potential bias and can meet the level of rigor often required by senior management, investors, or others responsible for providing the resources for additional development of the drug. Until recently, many if not most Phase II studies were too large and had too many clinical sites to make adaptive designs feasible.

Phase III studies are designed to test a hypothesis and must meet highest standards of statistical rigor. Also, in order to be acceptable to regulatory authorities, they must show a clinically meaningful benefit, and therefore must usually be large and with clinical endpoints that often require lengthy follow-up. Until recently, neither the statistical methodology nor logistic and technological tools existed to allow Phase III pivotal studies to be conducted with adaptive designs.

Also, importantly, each of the three phases has until recently been separate and distinct. Initially the Phase I study would be designed, conducted, and analyzed. Only after the analysis was complete would Phase II be designed, then conducted, and then analyzed. After the analysis of the Phase II study, the Phase III study would be designed, conducted, and analyzed.

Each phase was separate and distinct because at the time that modern clinical trials evolved, in the 1960s and 1970s, technology imposed significant limitations on the logistics of clinical trials. At that time, computers were not readily available, Internet did not exist, overnight package delivery did not exist, practical cell phones had not been invented, long distance phone calls were expensive, and even photocopiers were relatively new and expensive. These limitations required that clinical trials be conducted in distinct phases because it was very difficult to change the study once it was set in motion.

Clinical development had to be performed in "batch" style rather than in a continuous fashion because the cost of setup and change in the studies was very high.

As mentioned above, of all the phases, Phase I studies were conducted in a fashion the most similar to adaptive clinical trials. Because Phase I studies were often single-site studies with analytic facilities nearby, near-real-time data collection and analysis could be performed and adjustments made to the study rapidly. This was particularly true for early stage oncology studies, many of which have been adaptive for many years.

However, for Phase II and Phase III studies, the process took a long time. The protocols had to be written, reviewed, printed, and mailed to the sites. In an age of typewriters and mimeographs, the mere writing of the protocol took a long time. The typesetting and printing of the protocol also took a long time and was not inexpensive. Once set, changes to the protocol were not easily made. The case report forms (CRFs) had to be printed on special multiplicate paper. The typesetting had to be performed by professional typesetters or printers, since no personal computers existed. The proofs had to be reviewed and approved before the printing was done. The bulky CRFs had to be packaged and physically mailed to the sites. Drug filling and labeling took a significant amount of time since labeling had to be typeset and printed.

Once the study was started, it was a very laborious process to amend the study, since that meant handwriting the amendments, and having it typed, printed, and mailed. The CRFs had to be physically mailed to the sponsor, since faxing was neither widely available nor affordable and overnight mail did not exist. The time that was required to collect the CRFs, enter the data, check the data, and analyze the data—often with punch cards and mainframe computers or even manually—was very lengthy. It was laborious and slow to even track the studies before spreadsheets and project management software was available.

Given these limitations, clinical programs were conducted as start-stop processes. The decide-print-ship-initiate-collect data-process data-decide loop took months. The iterative loop between a decision to start one study and the next decision to start the next study could not usually occur in less than a year under the optimal circumstances, and usually took many years.

The era of discrete phase clinical trials is starting to draw to a close now with the dissolution of these practical logistic barriers. That multiyear cycle can now be reduced to months or sometimes weeks. Under the optimal circumstances, the gap between Phase I and Phase II or between Phase II and Phase III can be reduced to weeks or days. With modern seamless designs, the gap can be eliminated altogether in some cases.

A gradual shift away from the classic 3-phase paradigm has been building momentum for couple of decades. Sheiner's learn and confirm paradigm, discussed later, was a major turning point in the thinking about the structure of clinical development, and that paradigm itself is about to be eclipsed by modern adaptive design theories and techniques (Sheiner 1997).

The second barrier to adaptive clinical trials was lack of appropriate statistical methodology. In order to preserve statistical rigor in an adaptive trial, new statistical methods or adaptations of previous methods had to be invented. Classical study designs relied on relatively inflexible techniques that were poorly suited for adaptive designs. With the logistic challenges becoming more tractable, advances in statistical methodology have followed. In fact, as will be discussed later in the book, adaptive designs have exposed some of the fundamental weaknesses in classical statistical approaches to clinical trials and may lead eventually to wholesale revision of statistical approaches to both classical and adaptive trial designs.

In addition, the availability of affordable computers has allowed application of many of the new statistical methods. Many of the new statistical techniques are computationally demanding, and require a great deal of computing power. Simulations, for example, are often an important component of adaptive clinical trial designs, and simulations often require numerous calculations. Without modern microprocessors and computers, many of the new statistical methods would be impracticable.

1.3 Definition of Adaptive Clinical Trial

As with many other new fields, the definition of adaptive and flexible clinical trials has not been standardized. However, broadly speaking, adaptive clinical trials can be broadly defined as clinical studies that allow for changes in the design—patients, dosing, or other factors—during the course of the study, based on data generated during the study. In addition, these changes preserve the statistical integrity of the trial. Preserving statistical integrity means that the study can be considered to be hypothesis testing. This means that the results of the study can be used to support a conclusion that an intervention has a causal effect on the outcome. In other words, despite changing the study design in the course of the study, you can still conclude that the drug works if the results are positive.

This is important to note because it has always been possible to change a study while it is in progress, but not in such a way that the study still retains the ability to test the hypothesis.

Please note that the terminology of adaptive clinical trials is still evolving, and there are some differences in opinion about the term "adaptive clinical trials." There are many definitions for adaptive designs, with some being more congruent with each other than some others.

For example, the FDA defines adaptive design clinical study as follows:

"a study that includes a prospectively planned opportunity for modification of one or more specified aspects of the study design and hypotheses based on analysis of data (usually interim data) from subjects in the study. Analyses of the accumulating study data are performed at prospectively planned timepoints within the study, can be performed in a fully blinded manner or in an unblinded manner, and can occur with or without formal statistical hypothesis testing" (FDA 2010).

The EMA defines an adaptive trial as a study in which

"statistical methodology allows the modification of a design element (e.g. sample-size, randomization ratio, number of treatment arms) at an interim analysis with full control of the type I error" (Committee For Medicinal Products For Human Use 2010).

The term "flexible clinical trial" is often used as a synonym for adaptive clinical trial. However, in some publications, flexible is distinguished from adaptive clinical trials, in that flexible designs allow unplanned interim analysis of data and unplanned changes of study design on the fly, whereas adaptive designs are defined as designs where the potential adaptations and analysis are defined in advance. This is the definition I will follow in this book.

There are three sources of data that can drive changes or adaptations in the course of the study. The first source is data external to the study such as data from patients not enrolled in the study. The second source is blinded data from the study. The third source is unblinded data from the study.

The first type of adaptation, that based on external data, presents the least amount of statistical difficulty. In fact, most people would not consider those studies to be true adaptive studies. Many experts define true adaptive designs as ones that allow modification of the study based on data generated internally from the study itself, and exclude designs that are altered on basis of data generated externally from the study. This is because classical, non-Bayesian statistical methods are designed to be self-contained and in theory should not be affected by data external to the study.

An example of this first type of adaptation would be a change in the endpoint of a study based on results of a companion study. The companion study may yield results, for example, that suggest that an alternate endpoint would be more responsive to the drug. For example, let's imaging that two identical studies are being conducted on rheumatoid arthritis. The primary endpoint for both studies is ACR20, which is a response based on a constellation of physical symptoms and signs. As it happens, the first of the two studies is analyzed first and the primary endpoint is not met. However, prevention of joint erosion on x-ray, which is another way of assessing rheumatoid arthritis, yields a difference with a nominal p value of less than 0.05. A decision is taken to change the primary endpoint of the second study to joint erosion, but without breaking the blind of the second study. This type of change should not, in theory, change the statistical validity of the second study since no data from the second study are used to make the decision to alter the study endpoint.

Another example would be change in the dosage used in a study based on results of a separate pharmacokinetic study. For example, let's imagine that a study of an antidepressive drug is initiated with a 100-mg-per-day dose. Partway through the study, it is discovered that patients with a certain genetic variant of the cytochrome P_{450} gene metabolize the drug very quickly and that 200 mg per day would be more appropriate for those patients. The data comes from a separate study, not the study in question. A decision is made to increase the dose for the patients with that specific genetic variation. A decision to increase the sample size to compensate for lower efficacy in patients with the genetic variation who were already enrolled is also made. This type of adaptation should not jeopardize statistical rigor of the first study and can be instituted under the traditional non-adaptive clinical trial framework.

However, many of the principles that govern both internally derived and externally derived modifications overlap a great deal.

The second type of adaptation, that based on blinded data, offers minimal statistical risk if performed correctly. Examples would be change in sample size or endpoint based on blinded variance data from the study. For example, let's say a study of Down Syndrome patients is initiated with a sample size of 200 patients per arm. The sample size is based on prior published studies that indicate that standard deviation for the cognitive instrument, that serves as the primary endpoint in the study, has a standard deviation of 10. In the course of the study, it is discovered that the standard deviation for the instrument is actually 5. This standard deviation is calculated without breaking the blind. The sample size is reduced based on the correct standard deviation. Since the blind is not broken, statistical integrity is not jeopardized.

Other examples would include adaptations based on aggregate (combined data from all arms) clinical event rates, baseline characteristics, or discontinuation rates. For example, a study in myocardial infarction patients is undertaken with the assumption that the mortality will be 10%. However, it turns out that because of statin use and aggressive use of percutaneous intervention in the study by the cardiologists, the mortality is actually 5%. In the same study, the assumption is that 30% of the patients will have anterior myocardial infarction. However, it turns out that because another study is recruiting patients with anterior myocardial infarctions at many of the same clinical sites, the actual proportion of patients with anterior myocardial infarctions turns out to be 20%. And it happens that because the site coordinators at the sites are very experienced, the dropout rate is much lower than anticipated. So long as the blind is scrupulously maintained, the study can be adapted on the basis of these types of information without incurring much statistical risk.

The third type of adaptation, that based on unblinded data from the study, presents the greatest challenge. Changes in the study after the unblinded data have been viewed or assessed create significant risk of contamination of the study and can nullify the results. For example, let's say that a study of an anti-epileptic drug candidate is being conducted. The initial estimate of the magnitude of benefit is that the drug will reduce the frequency of seizures from 3 times a month to once a month. Partway through the study, the monitoring committee examines the unblinded data and it is discovered that the baseline seizure frequency is 4 times per month and the frequency of seizures in the treated group is 3 times per month. The study's sample size is increased on the basis of this information.

This type of adaptation can be done for a hypothesis testing study, but only under very controlled circumstances. Ideally, the changes and the parameters for the changes should be prespecified at the beginning of the study, and the unblinded data should be available to very few people, preferably only to an independent assessment committee. The ability to perform this type of adaptation is the most controversial and the most risky from a statistical viewpoint. However, with new methodologies and extremely meticulous clinical trial hygiene, these types of sophisticated adaptations can be done while preserving statistical integrity.

As mentioned earlier, not all studies that are changed during their course are adaptive studies. Changes to the study can occur by three processes. The first is a completely unplanned change to the study, one not meant to be an adaptive trial. For example, let's say a study is being conducted in diabetes patients comparing a drug candidate to an active comparator. Partway through the study, the comparator drug is withdrawn from market due to adverse events with the comparator drug. The trial may need to stop enrollment at that time even though there had been no intent to adapt the trial size. Another example would be a case where the sponsor arbitrarily decides to change the inclusion criteria. For example, a study can be conducted in multiple sclerosis patients with severe disease. The study enrolls very slowly and the sponsor decides to expand the entry criteria to patients with moderate disease in order to increase the enrollment rate. Another example might be a study where the original primary endpoint was to be 12-month mortality. It turns out that follow-up is very poor and 20% of the patients do not have 12-month follow-up visits. The primary endpoint is therefore amended to 6-month mortality. In these cases, these are not adaptive studies. They are non-adaptive studies that did not proceed as originally intended.

In a non-adaptive study, the blind must be completely maintained if the study results are not to be jeopardized. This is important because if the blind is broken, almost any study can be altered and manipulated to produce a false positive result. For example, let's say that in the third example above, the sponsor analyzes the unblinded 12-month mortality data and discovers that they are not statistically significant. The sponsor then analyzes the 3-month, 6-month, and the 9-month mortality data and discovers that the 6-month data are statistically significant. The sponsor then changes the primary endpoint to 6 months. This is unacceptable.

The second is an adaptive design where the analyses and adaptations for the entire study are planned in advance. We can call this a traditional adaptive clinical trial design. Many adaptive clinical studies prespecify how the design of the study will be altered as result of interim data, before the interim data are available or unblinded. In these studies, the study design is not fluid and cannot be changed at will at the discretion of the sponsor or the investigator. For example, let's say that a study of an asthma drug is being conducted. At the beginning of the study, it is prespecified that three interim analyses will be done. It is prespecified and documented at the beginning of the study that if the p value for the primary endpoint reaches 0.001 at the first interim analysis then the study will be terminated. It is prespecified at the beginning of the study that if the p value for the primary endpoint reaches 0.003 at the second interim analysis then the study will be terminated. And it is prespecified at the beginning of the study that if the p value for the primary endpoint reaches 0.01 at the third interim analysis then the study will be terminated. Both group sequential and so-called self-designing studies, described later in the book, fall into this second category. This is in contrast to a study where the number of analysis and the conditions for termination are not predefined.

An analogy might be a car driving on a road. A classical non-adaptive design prespecifies the route the driver must take. There can be no detour. There is only one route. A traditional adaptive design described above, allows two or more alternate routes. This type of adaptive design allows the driver to take a prespecified detour if there is an accident or a traffic jam on one route. Neither of these designs allows the driver the discretion to take the car on an un-prespecified route or off-road.

It should be noted that it is formally equivalent to prespecify adaptations at the beginning of the study or during the study so long as the blind is not broken before the adaptation. In general, although it is technically acceptable to prespecify the adaptations after the study has started so long as the data are unblinded, it is much better practice to prespecify before the initiation of the study, to minimize the possibility and perception of contamination. It is nontrivial to protect the blind once the study has started, and nontrivial to demonstrate that the blind has been protected.

The third, and more controversial type of adaptive design, prespecifies only one stage of the study at a time in advance, and leaves the study open for adaptation of almost any type after each interim analysis. Under this design, only the statistical weight and design of the immediate next must be prespecified. Once the interim is reached and the unblinded data are examined, the study design for the rest of the study can be modified almost at will, including the endpoint, sample size, and method of analysis.

As an example, let's say that a study of a new drug candidate is being conducted on patients with duodenal ulcers. The protocol prespecifies that an interim analysis will be done after 50 patients have been enrolled and

TABLE 1.1

Types of Study Changes and Adaptations

Source of Data	Unplanned (Non-Adaptive)	Prespecified Adaptive	Flexible Adaptive
External Source	Empiric changes Statistically valid	Empiric or adaptive changes Statistically valid	Empiric or adaptive changes Statistically valid
Blinded Internal Source	Empiric changes May be statistically valid	Adaptive changes Statistically valid	Adaptive changes Usually statistically valid
Unblinded Internal Source	Statistically invalid	Adaptive changes May be statistically valid	Adaptive changes May be statistically valid

that if the incidence of bleeding as determined by endoscopic examination is different enough between two groups to meet a p value of 0.01 or less, then the study will be terminated and the results will be positive. The study enrolls 50 patients and at the first interim analysis, the p value is not met. At that point, the unblinded data are examined, and the protocol is extended to another 50 patients. The amended protocol states that at that point, an interim analysis will be performed on the 100 patients and if the incidence of bleeding and non-bleeding ulcers is different enough to meet a p-value of 0.01 or less, then the study will be terminated and the results will be positive. At the second interim analysis, the endpoint is not met, and the protocol is extended by another 100 patients and a new endpoint of two or more bleeding ulcers is specified with a p value of 0.005 or less. And so on.

There is significant controversy about this type of novel adaptive technique. As mentioned above, some authors refer to this third type of adaptive design as flexible clinical trials. This type of trial is complex to design and to execute.

The three sources of data and three types of adaptations are summarized in Table 1.1

1.4 Precursors to Modern Adaptive Clinical Trials

As mentioned previously, adaptive clinical study designs are not completely novel. In many contexts, they have been used for decades.

For example, as mentioned above, Phase I trials have always lent themselves to adaptive designs because the patient numbers were limited and the studies were typically single-site studies. Also, the risks involved with potentially toxic untested agents in first-in-man studies are so great that there is a strong incentive to examine and understand the data from each dose level before escalation. In Phase I studies, it has been standard to administer a dose to a group of patients, analyze the data, and then determine the dose for the next group of patients.

Oncology studies have also been at the forefront of adaptive clinical designs. This is due to several factors. First, because oncology drugs are often tested to maximal toxicity, it is possible to generate meaningful amount of data in a small number of patients. For example, it is possible to specify the dose escalation based on the number of patients with dose limiting toxicity even if there are only three or six patients in each cohort. This is in contrast to other indications, such as depression, where the variability, placebo effect, and response rate may make it impossible to draw any conclusions based on a handful of patients. Second, for some types of cancer, oncology patients can be rare. This has made it necessary sometimes to use strategies such as adaptive trial designs, which maximize the data available from each patient. Third, the surrogate typically used in oncology studies lends itself to adaptive designs relatively well. For example, the classification of complete response/partial response/no response/progression of tumor, based on size, can be readily incorporated into a simple adaptive trial decision tree.

Data and safety monitoring boards (DSMB) have also made use of adaptive designs and statistical concepts for decades, albeit in a primitive fashion. Although in most cases, the extent of adaptation was limited to stopping the study or arms of the study and no more, the concepts developed for data and safety monitoring boards, including O'Brien–Fleming stopping boundaries, have laid some of the key groundwork for modern adaptive designs. These concepts, broadly accepted by statisticians, clinicians, and regulatory authorities, established the precedent that even within the framework of traditional non-Bayesian statistics, unblinded data could be examined by an independent committee and a decision based on that data could result in an alteration of the study. Importantly, these techniques established the precedent that even with such alterations the statistical integrity could be preserved. Once these precedents were set, it became a near certainty that as long as appropriate statistical techniques were developed to preserve the alpha (to keep the final aggregate p value below 0.05) other adaptations would be acceptable.

Covariate analysis is another type of well-accepted adaptation. It has been acceptable for many years to prespecify that the results of a study will be modified with covariate adjustments if the enrolled population is unbalanced in a particular fashion. For example, it is known that mortality after a myocardial infarction is affected by sex, size of the infarct, location of the infarct, and so on. It has been acceptable to prespecify in a study of myocardial infarction drugs, such as thrombolytics, that the mortality rate in the study could be adjusted on the basis of these known covariates. So, for instance, if the patients in one arm had higher mean infarct size, then the mortality rate in that arm could be adjusted downward before being compared to the other arm. It is not known at the beginning of the study what the covariate distribution will be in the study, and therefore covariate adjustment represents one type of simple adaptive design.

Other types of prespecified adaptations in the analysis of studies are also common. For example, handling of dropout data can be specified in advance, as can the analytic methods that will be used. For example, let's say a drug of ulcerative colitis is being studied. The primary endpoint is at 6 months but the sponsor believes that the dropout rate may be very high. The study can be designed so that alternate imputation strategies can be used depending on the dropout rate. If the dropout rate is below 10% at six months, "last observation carried forward" (LOCF) analysis would be used. This is a technique whereby the last available data point is used in patients with missing data. If the dropout rate is10% or higher, then the 3 month data would be used as the endpoint rather than the LOCF. And alternate data handling and analytic methods contingent on certain characteristics of the data set can be prespecified. For example, in the above study, it can be specified that if the distribution of the missing data is consistent across the two groups then one type of analysis be performed and if the distribution is unequal between the two groups then another type of analysis be performed.

Another common type of adaptation consists of run-in periods and enrichments (Temple 2006). A study population can be enriched on the basis of one of a number of factors, including pharmacodynamic or clinical response before randomization, tolerability to the drug, biomarker or surrogate response, and imaging. For example, a drug candidate is being studied in diabetes patients. Let's say that the drug is poorly tolerated, so that 20% of patients are expected to drop out within one week of starting the drug, but that those patients who tolerate the drug for a week are likely to tolerate the drug for the duration of the study. The study can be designed so that all patients receive the drug at the beginning of the study, and then at one week the patients can be randomized to continue the drug or to switch to placebo. This is an uncontroversial type of adaptive design that has been used in many studies.

Another common adaptation, which is so common that many people don't realize that it's an adaptation, is dose titration. Let's say that an enzyme replacement therapy is being tested in a genetic disease. The dose of the enzyme can be titrated on the basis of endogenous enzyme levels. Or as another example, an anticoagulant can be titrated on the basis of prothrombin time. These are adaptive designs in that the dose of the drug is not prespecified but rather is dependent on a variable that is collected in the course of the study.

On a slightly different tack, an important conceptual precursor to modern adaptive designs is the "learn and confirm" paradigm first proposed by Sheiner in 1997 (Sheiner 1997). By 1997, the logistic barriers to adaptive study designs had started to fade, and the weaknesses in the stepwise approach to clinical development were starting to become more evident. In this paradigm, Sheiner argued that the previous approach of hypothesis testing in each phase of clinical development was flawed. He argued that clinical trials should be divided into two broad categories. The first category would include all trials before Phase III, which he called the "learn" type of trial. He argued that the "learn" part of clinical studies should focus on the nature of the drug and its relationship to clinical effects should be characterized, rather than tested. These trials should be adaptive by their nature. The Phase III studies would represent the "confirm" type of trials. These trials would be non-adaptive and follow the traditional clinical trial design. This paradigm is discussed in more detail below.

1.5 New Enabling Technologies and Other Requirements for Adaptive Trials

Several new technologies have enabled the development of new adaptive designs.

The first is electronic data capture (EDC). Because the ubiquity of the internet, and the standardization associated with it, it is now possible to access data within hours or minutes of patient visits or of data generation. Tasks that used to take months—physically transporting CRFs to data management centers, processing the data, and collating the data—can now be done in seconds. In addition, data entry edit checks can be incorporated into EDC systems, reducing the time and effort required to clean the data. This rapid turnaround means that data for the adaptation can be collected and analyzed in a timely fashion. Without this speed, adaptive trials would be impossible because by the time the data analysis was available to enable the adaptation, the trial may be completed.

The second is affordable computer processing power and software. These have made practical computations and simulations necessary for some adaptive trial designs. As mentioned above, simulations are often necessary to design adaptive clinical trials. Importantly, coupled with EDC, this processing power also affords clinical trialists the ability to run iterative analysis— tables, listings, and graphs (TLGs)—quickly and as many times as desired. The processing power also makes real-time randomization possible, which enables adaptive allocation schemes. In addition, the modern computers make real-time project management of complex projects much more practical than when all the tracking had to be done manually.

The third is overnight delivery. With overnight delivery of drugs and material available to most places on the globe, it is now possible to quickly deliver material necessary to adapt the study. This is important because adaptations of the study often may necessitate replacement of a drug with different dosages if treatment arms are dropped or altered. In fact, without reliable worldwide overnight delivery, or at least express delivery, it would be virtually impossible to conduct modern adaptive studies that require changes in dosages or treatment arms.

The fourth is customized printing. Unlike in the past when typesetting and printing was a long and expensive process, customized printing (and low cost photocopying) allows adaptation of drug labels, protocols, and other study material in real time. Without inexpensive printers and printing, and without modern word processors that permit easy formatting, spellchecking, global find-and-replace, and other features we take for granted, even amending a protocol to change a few parameters would take an inordinate length of time.

The fifth is rapid communication systems, including Internet, interactive voice response systems (IVRSs), cell phones, digital radiology, and E-mail. These allow rapid communication and dissemination of changes in the protocols, rapid queries and resolutions, rapid changes in informed consent forms, and various other modifications. Gone are the days when the primary forms of communication over long distances were teletypes and mail.

The sixth is advances in rapid analytics of biochemical and chemical samples. Coupled with overnight shipping and other advances enumerated above, this allows rapid turnaround of biological samples and incorporation of the data into the decision-making process. Modern analytic methods are flexible and rapid, and are usually computerized. Liquid chromatography–mass spec techniques are highly accurate. Polymerase chain reactions are exquisitely sensitive. Automated cell counters and chemical analyzers can process a large number of samples quickly and inexpensively. In some cases, on-site analysis can be performed with benchtop machines that are highly accurate and rapid, allowing real-time availability of results.

The above advances, along with new statistical methods discussed later in this book, have opened the doors wide for adaptive clinical trials. Of course, in addition to the new enabling technologies, certain other requirements are necessary or highly desirable for adaptive clinical trials, such as regulatory acceptability and operational/executional processes that are re-engineered for adaptable clinical trials. These other requirements are discussed later in the book.

1.6 Rationale for Adaptive Clinical Trials

There are several important rationales for using adaptive clinical designs. While traditional studies still have an important role in clinical development, in many cases adaptive studies are much better suited.

The most important rationale for using adaptive clinical trials is the ethical rationale. All clinical trials, by their very nature, expose patients to risk.

The risks fall into two categories. First, no drug is completely safe. Even a well characterized drug exposes patients to risks they would not otherwise incur. However, many drugs in clinical trials are not well characterized, and the known and the unknown risks for patients exposed to those drugs can be very high.

Second, all patients in clinical trials incur the risk that they may be deprived of a superior therapy because the arm in which they are enrolled is less effective than the other arm, or not effective at all. All trials require equipoise, or some degree of uncertainty as to which of the arms is superior, because otherwise it is unethical to conduct the clinical trial. Because of this, patients always run the risk that they will not receive the best therapy.

Clearly, it is unethical to expose patients to any more risk than is absolutely necessary. Adaptive designs generally lower the number of patients potentially exposed to unsafe or ineffective drugs and raise the number exposed to safe and/or effective drugs. Adaptive designs often allow early termination of ineffective arms or doses. Adaptive designs also permit early termination of studies that appear futile or appear to show very high levels of difference between the two arms.

As adaptive studies become more feasible and acceptable to regulatory authorities, it is not unlikely that traditional clinical trials will be considered to be unethical except in a limited set of circumstances, because by their very design, traditional studies enroll more patients than actually necessary.

The second and third reasons for using adaptive clinical trials are economic. Clinical trials using adaptive designs, by lowering the sample sizes, usually reduce the cost of drug development. By allowing early termination of futile studies, they also reduce costs. In addition, continuous/seamless designs and adaptive designs shorten development timelines substantially which also reduces costs. Simply by eliminating the interval between Phase I and Phase II and between Phase II and Phase III, seamless designs can reduce the total development time for a drug by one or two years. Given that the opportunity cost a single day's delay in approval of a drug that is anticipated to reach peak market sales of a billion dollars is several million dollars, this reduction in time is clearly very valuable.

The fourth and fifth reasons are scientific. Adaptive designs, if properly used, can provide more information from clinical trials. For example, the designs may better define a dose response curve or better define the relationship between demographic factors and response. There can be more data points, and the data points can be collected in such a way in adaptive studies so that more data points are collected at doses or in patients that are more informative. Adaptive designs can also increase the likelihood of success for the study in certain cases, and may yield a better drug in terms of dose, dosing, or subgroup definition. In some cases, adaptive clinical trials can produce information that is simply not possible to collect from a traditional non-adaptive study.

1.7 Learn and Confirm

Although the traditional divisions of clinical trials are between Phase I, Phase II, and Phase III, these are somewhat artificial distinctions, driven largely by pragmatic needs. They define the way information is collected and conclusions are drawn in chunks or batches. Each batch is represented by a study or a protocol.

On a more logical, conceptual level, most clinical trials can be divided into descriptive and hypothesis-testing trials. In fact, a better way of thinking about clinical development of a drug is not by phases or clinical trials but by a flow of data and information. Traditional clinical trials are analogous to a bucket brigade, transferring water bucket by bucket. Adaptive studies are analogous to a fire hose, which can be turned on and off at will. Where the clinical information is generated is important, but much more important is the totality of information generated. However, for purposes of keeping to conventional terminology, I will discuss the flow of information in the framework of clinical trials.

About ten years ago, Sheiner published an important paper delineating the difference between descriptive, or what he called learning phase trials, and hypothesis testing, or what he called confirming trials in Figure 1.1 (Sheiner 1997). Other terminology for descriptive trials includes exploratory, Phase I, Phase II, and Phase IIa. Other terminology for hypothesis-testing trials include adequate and well-controlled, pivotal, and Phase III.

In his paper, Sheiner argued that while the purpose of a confirmatory trial is to test a hypothesis, and the output of the study is a binary answer, earlier stage trials are designed to explore and learn the response curves associated with therapies. He correctly recognized that the non-confirmatory studies, while often designed in a similar fashion as the confirmatory studies, actually have a different purpose. It therefore stands to reason that the design of such studies should be different from the confirmatory studies.

Proper design of the descriptive or "learn" type of studies is important for several reasons. First, the information from the learning period is very important because it allows proper design of the confirmatory study. Collecting and characterizing as much information as possible about the dose response, toxicity curve, subgroups' difference in response and adverse events, PK/PD characteristics, and other factors all improve the likelihood of success in the confirmatory studies if the information is utilized effectively.

And, as he rightly points out, clinicians who will be using the drug also often need that information. Simply knowing that a drug works is insufficient to maximize the utility of the drug after approval. It is very well to know that the drug works, but the practitioner also needs to know how the drug works, in whom, and in what fashion. The physician needs information about which patients are likely to experience side effects, which concomitant medications may be inadvisable, whether dosage adjustments may be

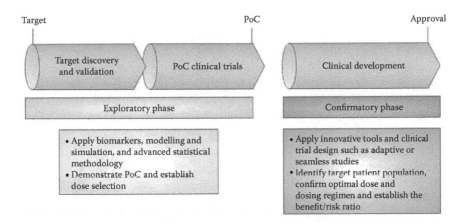

FIGURE 1.1
Learn and confirm paradigm. Reprinted from Orloff, J. "The future of drug development: Advancing clinical trial design." In *Nature Reviews Drug Discovery* 8, 949–957 (December 2009). With permission.

needed in renal failure patients, and a multitude of additional pieces of data. Some of the questions Sheiner highlighted include

- What is an appropriate initial dose for my particular patient?
- How soon will intended effect start?
- How long will it last? Will tolerance develop?
- What happens if my patient misses some doses?
- What are the chances that the initial dose will have to be altered?
- What do I follow to see if it needs to be altered?
- How do I alter it? Do I wait 1 week, 2 weeks, 3 weeks? Do I then suggest a big increment or a small one?

The framework he suggested is the therapeutic–response curve, shown in Figure 1.2. Patient prognostic factors such as age or disease are on one axis, the drug dose or regimen on the second axis, and the benefit on the z-axis. For any given patient, there is an optimum dose that in this case is the same for everyone but in reality varies from patient to patient and corresponding benefit level.

Sheiner discusses three areas where there are substantial differences between the two types of trials: assignment (randomization, blinding, dosing, and demographics of enrolled patients), observation (prognostic factors, exposure, outcome), and analysis (hypothesis testing vs. estimation).

When a confirmatory trial is designed, the doses are usually fixed and wide apart (in other words, the control arm usually is receiving placebo or dose of zero). There is usually no adaptation of the dose, and there is usually one active dose and one placebo dose. If there is more than one active dose,

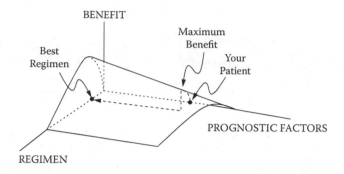

FIGURE 1.2
A dose–response curve for response can be plotted together with the dose–response curve for toxicity, and the two can help define the area of maximal separation. Reprinted with permission from Sheiner, L.B. "Learning versus confirming in clinical drug development." *Clin. Pharmacol. Ther.* 275–291 (1997).

the doses tend to be well separated. This is because the goal of the confirmatory trial is to establish a difference between the dose groups.

Confirmatory trials also usually are blinded, and the patients are randomized, since both of these are important in protecting statistical validity. Blinding and randomization, however, reduce flexibility of the trial and reduces the amount of information that can be collected.

In confirmatory trials, the patients chosen are a homogeneous group, which helps increase the statistical power. The inclusion and exclusion criteria clearly define the target population to be enrolled, and it is not advisable to change the criteria during the study. This is because the more homogeneous the population is, the less variability, and the greater the power of the study to detect a difference in response, at least using traditional statistical methods.

Also, in a confirmatory study, observation is focused on the primary endpoint. Secondary endpoints may be collected, but the goal of the trial is not to maximize the amount of information collected. Confirmatory studies are often large and complex. Any additionally extraneous collected information increases the cost of the study substantially and is generally considered to be poor practice.

And of course the final analysis is hypothesis-testing and usually frequentist. The goal of a confirmatory trial is to establish causality between the intervention and response.

For a learning study, on the other hand, you want to test multiplicity of doses, and you want to test doses clustered together near the ideal dose so that you build a complete and detailed picture of the dose–response curve. The goal is not to show a difference between doses. The goal in a learning trial is to define as well as possible the dose response, particularly the dose response at the anticipated therapeutic dose.

In a learning trial, the goal is to enroll as wide variety of patients as possible to get a richer picture of the covariates that impact response. A wide variety of sex, age, genetic profiles, weight, and other demographic factors can and often should be tested to determine if there is an impact on PK, PD, safety, efficacy, or other outcome variable. Other variabilities, such as concomitant medications and stage of the disease, should also be assessed if possible, within limits of practicality and resource constraints.

In a learning study, the goal is also to capture multiple pharmacological and clinical outcomes. Rather than focusing only on the primary outcome, obtaining information about a multitude of endpoints and measures is advisable. This allows a fuller understanding and characterization of the effect of the drug, which allows for optimal design of the subsequent trials.

The analysis of a learning trial is more complicated than for a confirmatory trial because in order to understand a multitude of data from widely disparate populations, it is usually necessary to use mathematical modeling to display and synthesize the results. The results are not binary as in a confirmatory trial. Binary answers are easy to interpret. In a learning trial, the answer is not a yes/no but rather a description of the relationship between the drug, variable such as demographic factors, and response.

Modeling refers to the process of plotting the data on a graph and using mathematical regression analysis to come up with a curve that best fits the data. There is sparse amount of data at any one point, or for any one subgroup. However, by mathematically analyzing the data at multiple points, a general description of the relationship between the variables and outcomes can be derived. The curve describing this relationship can be on a two-dimensional graph, three-dimensional graph, or a multidimensional representation.

Modeling is helpful in clinical development, but has some significant drawbacks. One of the most important is that with one set of data, many different models can be constructed because the assumptions used in the modeling play a critical role in how the results turn out. Because of this, the modeling is rarely conclusive and is open to multiple interpretations.

Sheiner also argued that the relationship between pharmacokinetics/ exposured and clinical outcome should be used to understand responses. In other words, rather than just relying on the dose–response relationship, he, like many pharmacologists, regarded the relationship between exposure and response as more important. While intuitively, this makes sense, in that a drug cannot exert its effects if it is not absorbed, it is inaccurate. This is an important and common fallacy that should be thoroughly understood.

Sheiner is wrong in his assertion, because significant confounding can occur in exposure–response analysis. For instance, factors that reduce or increase absorption of the drug can play an important role in the prognosis of the patient in many cases and the exposure–response relationship. For example, for an anti-diarrheal drug, the patients with the worst prognosis may also happen to have the poorest drug absorption and the exposure and prognosis may be correlated but not because of efficacy of the drug. Therefore, the existence of a relationship between drug exposure and an outcome does not mean that the drug caused the outcome. There might be a third independent factor that affected the exposure and the outcome in a similar fashion.

Of course, learning trials can be performed without adaptation. However, learning trials are ideally suited for adaptive designs. The flexibility of adaptive clinical trial design allows rich exploration of the parameters of relevance to learning trials. For example, because adaptive designs allow changes in design during the study, it can be used to explore the dose–response curve in an efficient fashion, collecting additional data where there are gaps in data, and collecting finer resolution data near the inflexion points.

1.8 Classification and Terminology of Adaptive Clinical Studies

Because the field of adaptive designs is new, terminology is still shifting. In general, adaptive study designs are those that incorporate new data in the course of the study to make changes in the study, as defined above. The changes can affect almost any facet of the study, including the list below taken from FDA's guidance document on adaptive studies (FDA 2010).

- study eligibility criteria (either for subsequent study enrollment or for a subset selection of an analytic population)
- randomization procedure
- treatment regimens of the different study groups (e.g., dose level, schedule, duration)
- total sample size of the study (including early termination)
- concomitant treatments used
- planned schedule of patient evaluations for data collection (e.g., number of intermediate timepoints)
- timing of last patient observation and duration of patient study participation)
- primary endpoint (e.g., which of several types of outcome assessments, which timepoint of assessment, use of a unitary versus composite endpoint or the components included in a composite endpoint)
- selection and/or order of secondary endpoints
- analytic methods to evaluate the endpoints (e.g., covariates of final analysis, statistical methodology, Type I error control)

Adaptive clinical trials encompass a wide field that is expanding rapidly. The various designs are fully explored in detail later in the book but briefly summarized here. The simplest studies are individual sequential designs, also known as fully sequential designs. These studies incorporate analysis of data after each patient or each data point, and adapt the next dose or patient treatment accordingly. Group sequential designs are designs that incorporate one or more interim analysis and can lead to termination of one or more arms of the study. Modern true adaptive designs incorporate multiple analyses, sometimes on a continual basis, and can lead to changes in almost any design parameter.

Seamless clinical trials are trials that combine more than one traditional phase of clinical development. For example, a study that combines both Phases II and III into one study without a gap between the end of Phase II and the start of Phase III would be a seamless clinical trial. As the FDA points out, the distinction between non-seamless and seamless trials is semantic from a regulatory stance but for sponsors, the distinction is important because the operational and financial implications can be different between the two types of trials

Bayesian clinical trials or Bayesian analyses are related to adaptive designs. Bayesian statistics rely on epistemological principles that are distinct from traditional frequentists. Adaptive designs by their very nature rely on Bayesian-type changes in the conduct of the study but the conclusions are usually based on non-Bayesian statistics. Bayesian analysis is discussed later in the book.

1.9 Non-Adaptive Study Designs

Sometimes misclassified as adaptive designs, unplanned changes to the study implemented because of data external to the study, because of data from the study, or because of logistics, are not adaptive designs. An example is the Provenge Phase III study in which the primary endpoint was altered based on the results of another Phase III study that completed earlier. This was not an adaptive design because there was no prior plan to potentially change the endpoint before the unexpected results were seen in the first study. Another example is change in the exclusion criteria, prohibiting patients with cardiovascular risk factors because in the course of a study an imbalance in myocardial infarction rate is detected. Another example is broadening of the inclusion criteria because enrollment is unexpectedly slow.

1.10 Limitations of Adaptive Clinical Trials

There are several limitations and risks of adaptive clinical trials. Some of these limitations should eventually become less problematic as clinical trialists, regulatory agencies, ethics committees, and sponsors/site personnel gain more experience with adaptive studies and as methods to address the issues are developed.

The first risk is that because logistic, statistical, and operational processes for adaptive clinical trials are new, there might be unanticipated mistakes and errors in the operational aspects of the trial. Currently, the number of people who have successfully executed modern adaptive trials is limited. As discussed later, the operational challenges for adaptive studies can be quite significant. In particular, maintaining the blind is non-trivial even under the best circumstances and inadvertent unblinding may easily occur in the course of an adaptive study. Also, the multiple changes to the protocol and procedures as well as extensive customization of each site and/or patient can present major challenges.

In addition, regulatory authorities may be uncomfortable with some types of adaptive designs. Regulatory authorities are not generally amenable to accepting controversial statistical techniques, and there is still significant debate within the statistical community about some of the techniques used in certain types of adaptive clinical trials. In particular, the debate is heated regarding what types of statistical analyses are and are not acceptable for preserving the alpha. Whenever unblinded data are being used for decision making in the midst of a study, the techniques for compensating for the decisions may not adequately address the risk for Type I error. Also, by their very nature, adaptive studies are slightly less statistically efficient than fixed studies. This is discussed later in the book. However, the loss of this efficiency is usually more than made up by non-statistical efficiencies afforded by adaptive designs. These issues should also resolve over time as more experience is gained and statisticians reach greater consensus.

Another potential limitation, which applies to any sort of streamlined development process, is that less extraneous data are generated. For the most part, this is an advantage, but it may lead to some potential adverse effects of the drug not being discovered because the data set may often be smaller and more focused for adaptive studies. An advantage of adaptive trials is that fewer patients need to be studied. At the same time, however, the smaller the number of patients, the less likely it is that a rare adverse event will be detected. Also, because some adaptive study designs are extremely parsimonious, and yield positive or negative answers with minimal numbers of patients, they may not give a good estimate of the magnitude of the effect. The sponsor may know that the drug works, but may not know how well it works, because the trial changed so many parameters.

1.11 Performance Criteria for Well Designed Clinical Trials

There is great interest in adaptive trial designs, but also intense debate. How can we determine if adaptive clinical trials offer an advantage? To address this question, it is helpful to examine characteristics that distinguish a good clinical trial from a bad one, and assess adaptive clinical trials from that context.

As with any scientific experiment, the first criterion for a clinical trial is: are the results accurate? This is sometimes referred to as internal validity. A well-designed clinical trial should render clear and accurate assessment of the hypothesis being tested. When the null hypothesis is false, the study should reject it (avoid Type I error), and when it is the study should not reject it (avoid Type II error).

When Type I and II errors are avoided, then the results are accurate and internal validity is achieved. When a Type I or Type II error results, then the results are not accurate and internal validity is not met. In other words, the trial results are wrong. The trial shows statistically significant difference between the two arms when in fact the intervention has no effect, or the trial shows no difference when in fact the intervention is effective.

Inaccurate results sometime arise because of poor study design. In other cases, back luck or random chance leads to inaccurate results. Clinical trials are not exact, and there is always the effect of random variability that can skew the results.

Worse than an inaccurate result is an uninterpretable result. This can be due to poor study design. For example, perhaps the study was under-powered, did not test a high enough dose, or was terminated too early. It may also be due to poor quality data, because of missing data, patient dropouts, or unreliable measurements. It may also be due to failure to minimize bias, such that the results are not reliable. Unfortunately, one of the most common causes for uninterpretable results is poor study design.

In order for a study to render valid conclusions, it must be free of bias. Bias is an error that changes the result of a study in a spurious manner. Bias can be classified into several categories (Table 1.2).

Systematic bias is a study-wide error that affects both the control and active arms equally. They include biases such as training effect, better health care due to patients being in the study, and time bias. For example, if a study requires multiple treadmill tests, the patients may become better conditioned over time simply because they get used to the treadmill. All of these can affect the generalizability of the study, but because they affect both control and treated arms equally, they do not usually affect the ability to draw conclusions regarding the differences between the arms (internal validity).

Differential bias affects arms of a study unequally and does represent a threat to internal validity of a study because such biases affect the apparent efficacy of the treatment. One important differential bias is differences in baseline characteristics. For example, if healthier patients are assigned to the treatment arm, they may have better outcomes simply because they are healthier at the beginning of the study. Randomization, stratification, and, in some cases, multivariate adjustments can address the bias from imbalances in baseline characteristics at the beginning of the study.

TABLE 1.2

Types of Biases

Systematic Bias (e.g., training effect)	Differential Bias		
	Bias at Initiation (e.g., imbalance in demographic factors)	**Bias During Trial**	
		Bias due to effect of the drug (e.g., greater efficacy not requiring symptomatic medications)	Bias due to knowledge of treatment assignment (e.g., more exertion on treadmill)

Another differential bias is differences that exist not at the initiation of the study but arise during the course of the study. Examples include differences in how the patients are assessed, placebo effect, differences in dropout rates, etc. For example, a physician may unconsciously score the patients in the treatment arm better when assessing the outcome because he believes strongly that the drug works.

Adaptive clinical trials, when properly designed, maintain the level of Type I error at acceptable levels under the frequentist rubric (p value of 0.05 or less). In many instances, it can reduce Type II error levels significantly below that that can be achieved with conventional designs. In other instances, it takes advantage of Bayesian techniques simply unavailable to conventional designs and arguably results in better accuracy.

As for other applied sciences, the second performance criterion for clinical trials is: are the results of the study useful? Usefulness is comprised of three parts. First, positive results are usually more useful than negative results, so the study should be optimized for likelihood of a positive result. Of course, positive results are only useful if the net benefit is meaningful. For example, it is not useful to improve one symptom of a disease while worsening another. So the question being posed by the trial must be well formed. Also, the study should be designed so that the results are applicable to real-life patients, and of use to the practicing clinician.

In most instances, a safe and effective therapy is more useful to the clinician than one that is not. Therefore, demonstrating that a therapy is safe and effective for a disease is more desirable than demonstrating that it isn't. Therefore a clinical trial design should maximize the likelihood of positive study results. A study that is well designed, in addition to yielding accurate results, also poses the right question. For example, a study looking at the impact on 30-day mortality of 100 mg of a certain drug in severe sepsis patients may yield an accurate result that it has no impact. However, it may be that 200 mg of the drug in moderate sepsis patients has a beneficial impact on 60-day mortality. Selecting the right patient population, the right dose, and the right endpoint has a critical impact on the likelihood of success.

Adaptive designs often increase the likelihood of success. This is largely because they allow better calibration of study parameters such as sample size to reality, and rely less on assumptions,

It is important that the question have construct validity. For instance, if the purpose of the study is to determine whether a thrombolytic drug has a beneficial effect on myocardial infarction patients, including the incidence of re-ischemia and congestive heart failure without including death as part of a composite endpoint might lead to inappropriate conclusions. This is because congestive heart failure and re-ischemia rates might increase even when the therapy is providing a benefit. Patients who would have died might live but with congestive heart failure. Similarly, measuring myelitis without accounting for renal failure in lupus patients may yield the erroneous conclusion that the drug is beneficial when in fact it merely shifts one manifestation of the disease to another.

Adaptive trials have neither advantages nor disadvantages compared to conventional studies with regard to proper formation of the question.

The goal of a clinical trial is to generate knowledge about whether an intervention can help patients with a disease. The results must be useful in clinical practice—have external validity and be actionable. It must have external validity in that the types of patients who are enrolled should not be so specific and homogeneous that the results seen in those patients would be different from those in clinical practice. The characteristics of the patients, intervention, and outcome in the clinical trial must be close enough to clinical practice in order to be transferable to everyday practice. In addition, the results of the clinical trial must be actionable in that the drug should be given in a fashion that would be practicable in the real world, and the patients must be treated in a similar fashion as they would be in real practice. For example, administration of a drug six times a day would not be practicable in clinical practice.

There is significant amount of controversy about external validity of adaptive trials. Specifically, the issue is whether the results are interpretable and understandable to the practicing clinician. This concern is often justified. In an adaptive trial, the patient population and/or the null hypothesis can be altered, sometimes multiple times, in the course of the study. In such cases, it makes the study hard to interpret because it may be difficult to identify the specific population that stands to benefit, or which outcome actually improved. While conventional study designs can also face similar issues if the protocol is amended in the course of the study, the problem is magnified with adaptive designs. Unfortunately, the current adaptive techniques do not fully address this concern.

Because a clinical trial enrolls human subject, the third and most important criterion is: does the trial protect patient safety and is it ethical? Does it limit risk to subjects by involving the fewest number of patients necessary? Clinical trials must be designed to minimize any potential harm to the patients.

Adaptive designs can sometimes expose patients to greater danger if improperly designed, but in general, they are much more parsimonious and do a better job of enrolling fewer patients in ineffective or less-safe arms. There is no doubt that adaptive trials offer an advantage from an ethical viewpoint.

In addition, a well-designed study yields not just the right answer but also the maximum quantity and quality of data while utilizing the least amount of resources. A well-designed clinical trial enrolls the fewest number of patients necessary to answer the scientific question or hypothesis being tested. In this way, fewer patients are exposed to risk inherent in all clinical trials.

In addition to the performance criteria outlined above, the clinical trial should also be feasible. From a practical viewpoint, a trial should be designed so that it can be enrolled, the patients can be compliant with the requirements of the trial, measurements can be taken, and so on. If a trial cannot be conducted in a real world, it is of little value. Sometimes the protocol will have unreasonably narrow inclusion criteria, specify very difficult requirements (such as prohibition of common concomitant medications), or require logistically difficult procedures (such as FACS analysis within 12 hours of blood collection). In such cases, the trial will often need to be amended or in some cases terminated early. In either case, the validity of the study is affected. Even in cases short of requiring an amendment, the study can become plagued with errors and protocol violations. There are also logistics considerations—for example, it may become prohibitively expensive because of the procedures required.

Adaptive designs have almost an insurmountable advantage over conventional trials with regard to parsimony. They are much more efficient than conventional trials. They also tend to lower cost and timelines significantly. With regard to feasibility, however, adaptive trials are more difficult to conduct well and are relatively new.

Apart from the above performance criteria, there is an important fundamental question about adaptive designs that is not yet fully resolved. Adaptive designs can be powerful, but the statistical techniques are still in the process of being developed. The demands being placed on conventional statistical techniques are straining the conventional frequentist statistical methods to the breaking point. Currently, this strain is being manifested as debate about the validity and integrity of adaptive techniques. Validity and integrity are sometimes defined differently but as mentioned before, internal validity means that the conclusions from a study represent the truth; external validity means that the results of a trial can be extrapolated to the broader patient population as a whole, and integrity means that the blind and other statistical formalities have been properly maintained. Because the traditional statistical techniques are poorly suited for adaptive designs, it may not be possible to address the needs of adaptive clinical trials within the standard statistical framework. Eventually, the choice may come down to rejecting adaptive designs as violating the current statistical paradigm or revising the fundamental basis of clinical trial statistics.

The intense debate about adaptive designs and their ability to meet the validity and integrity requirements is still raging. When all is said and done, and the statisticians have had full vetting of the techniques, it may turn out that adaptive designs fail these tests. However, the advantages offered by adaptive designs are formidable, both scientifically and ethically, and it is possible or perhaps likely that if something has to give, the current fundamental statistical basis of clinical trials will make way for the new methodologies.

The above description of the key performance criteria for clinical trials is adapted from (Chin and Lee 2008).

1.12 Evolving Regulatory Environment for Adaptive Clinical Trials

Adaptive clinical trials, especially those meant to serve as pivotal hypothesis-confirming trials, must meet the requirements of regulators if they are to lead to new drug approvals. Regulators, including the FDA and EMA, have expressed cautious optimism that adaptive clinical trials can be a useful tool. FDA has published a draft guideline on Adaptive Clinical Trials for Drugs and Biologics (FDA 2010) and a final Guidance for the Use of Bayesian Statistics in Medical Device Clinical Trials (FDA 2010). EMA has issued several documents on adaptive clinical trials, including a report on the EMEA-EFPIA Workshop on Adaptive Designs in Confirmatory Clinical Trials (EMA 2010).

In 2006, Scott Gottlieb, the Deputy Commissioner for Medical and Scientific Affairs at the FDA, gave a speech at the Conference on Adaptive Trial Designs, promoting the use of adaptive designs. This speech created quite a bit of excitement, but like many other large organizations, FDA has moved with deliberate speed since then, reflecting a divergence of views on the topic within the agency. For drugs and biologics, the FDA has made the following points:

1. Non-pivotal studies (studies that are not intended to be "adequate and well controlled" [A&WC studies]) may use adaptive design freely. The FDA is much more concerned about validity of adaptive designs for A&WC studies.

2. Traditional adaptive designs that clearly preserve the alpha, such as group sequential designs, pose no regulatory problems.

3. Adaptive designs that rely on blinded data, such as variance or other "nuisance" parameters pose, no regulatory problems. This is the case even if the blinded data lead to changes in the primary endpoint or the analytic method for the primary endpoint.

4. Adaptation based on data external to the study is acceptable, and in fact the FDA does not consider such studies to be adaptive designs.

5. New flexible designs that allow modification of study designs after the interim unblinded analysis may or may not be valid and FDA will view them cautiously. However, they do not rule out the potential for utilizing such designs, especially in circumstances where other designs may not be sufficient.

   Dose-finding adaptive designs may in some special circumstances be appropriate for pivotal studies, although FDA sees more of a role for them in Phase II studies.

   The FDA regards adaptive randomization with some caution, particularly in cases where it may result in an imbalance in patient characteristics among the groups as this can introduce a bias, but may be open to it if used carefully.

   Changes in sample size after an unblinded interim analysis is also regarded with some caution by the FDA, and they emphasize that alpha inflation must be avoided scrupulously.

   Similarly, changes in the inclusion and exclusion criteria or in the endpoint are also regarded cautiously, and the FDA points out that interpretation of studies incorporating such changes can be challenging.

   Adaptation of noninferiority study can be done, but the FDA points out that unblinded analysis may not be necessary in most cases, and that the changes in the noninferiority margin cannot be changed.

6. A single adaptive study with multiple stages cannot by itself fulfill the replication requirement for drug approval. It is still considered to be a single study. The presumption, though not stated in the guidance, is that the study must then meet the standard requirement for non-replicated studies if it is to support approval without an additional pivotal study, namely p value of 0.00125 or less.

7. The FDA cautions that since adaptive designs can be so much more parsimonious in terms of study size and rapid dose escalation, patient safety may be jeopardized unless extreme care is taken to safeguard patient safety.

8. They also note that modeling may be useful in planning some types of adaptive studies.

9. Special protocol assessments (SPA) may be problematic with adaptive designs because it is difficult for the FDA to commit to such open ended designs with an SPA.

10. Protocols for adaptive studies should include certain elements:
    - Summary of information about the drug
    - Explanation of why adaptive design is appropriate

- Description of adaptations envisioned, assumptions behind the adaptations, statistical techniques, methods for assessing outcome, and calculations of treatment effect
- Impact of the adaptations on the statistical parameters, especially the alpha but also power and confidence intervals
- Computer simulations of the adaptations and its impact on the statistical parameters and bias, and all branch points
- Computer program used for the simulation
- Analytic techniques to be used
- Written procedures and charters for the personnel carrying out the study and performing the interim analysis, including how firewalls will be established and maintained

11. Great care must be taken to insure that blind and study integrity is maintained. SOPs specific to adaptive designs must be in place, and clinical research organizations that do not have experience in adaptive studies may not be able to execute the study properly.

The last point is worth emphasizing. As will be discussed later, adaptive studies are not easy to operationalize, and there is a reasonably high risk that the study integrity may be compromised. As Bob Temple, Associate Director for Medical Policy from the FDA, commented in 2006 at the Adaptive Designs Workshop, we should also remember that adaptive design is no substitute for good drug development principles. Adaptive designs should not be used as a replacement for good planning and science.

The EMA has been somewhat more lukewarm than the FDA to the concept of adaptive clinical trials. It published "Reflection Paper on Methodological Issues in Confirmatory Clinical Trials with Flexible Design and Analysis Plan" in 2007 that outlines its position on adaptive clinical trials. Its views are as follows.

1. It can be challenging to maintain the integrity of an adaptive clinical trial. Nonetheless, the integrity is extremely important.
2. Group sequential designs with fixed or prespecified stopping rules for interim analysis are acceptable.
3. EMA cautions against risks posed by overrunning. Overrunning refers to patients who are not included in the interim analysis but are already enrolled in the study, who may contribute to the endpoint once all data has been collected. The data from those patients can affect final results and may change the conclusions compared to the interim analysis.
4. Changes in the design of a Phase III study after it has started are strongly discouraged. If changes are made, then the two stages of the

study before and after the changes must be homogeneous enough to allow meaningful analysis.

5. Sample size re-estimation is not encouraged but acceptable if performed carefully.

6. Changes to the primary endpoint in the midst of a study are not acceptable.

7. Group sequential methods dropping groups at the interim analysis can be performed with caution.

8. Switching between noninferiority and superiority can be performed with caution, particularly if the switch is from noninferiority to superiority.

9. Randomization ratio can be changed during the study.

10. Phase II/III seamless studies cannot be used in lieu of a conventional Phase III because it doesn't fulfill the requirement that a Phase III study be a confirmatory trial.

In addition, the FDA has issued a guidance on Bayesian statistics in medical device trials (FDA 2010). In it, adaptive designs are considered, and though specifics are lacking, the agency appears very accommodating to adaptive studies performed for devices using Bayesian design (FDA 2010).

In summary, the regulatory authorities are comfortable with adaptive designs in the non-pivotal or non-confirmatory clinical trials. They are cautiously optimistic about the use of adaptive designs in pivotal clinical studies designed to result in approval of a drug.

1.13 Regulatory Guidance from the FDA

The FDA has issued some specific guidance on how the sponsor should interact with the FDA with regard to adaptive clinical trials during the planning, conduct, and reporting of the study, as outlined in the excerpt below from (FDA 2010).

> The purpose and nature of the interactions between a study sponsor and FDA varies with the study's location (stage) within the drug development program. The increased complexity of some adaptive design studies and uncertainties regarding their performance characteristics may warrant earlier and more extensive interactions than usual. This section discusses general principles on interactions between sponsors and FDA with regard to the use of adaptive designs 1585 in a development program.

A. Early and Middle Period of Drug Development

FDA's review of an exploratory study protocol is usually focused upon the safety of the study participants, and does not typically scrutinize the protocol as closely for design elements related to assessment of pharmacologic activity, efficacy, and strength of inferences. As resources allow, however, FDA might review exploratory protocols to consider the relevance of the information being gathered to guide the design of later studies (e.g., do the doses being examined seem reasonable for early efficacy evaluations; are the endpoints or biomarkers being examined reasonable for the stage of drug development).

Review comments from the FDA on the adaptive design features in exploratory protocols will generally be less formal than for late stage drug development studies. Sponsors who have specific questions about the adaptive design elements in an exploratory study should seek FDA feedback either by identifying the specific issues, questions, and the requested feedback in the submission containing the protocol, or by requesting a meeting to discuss specific questions.

Discussion of the plans for an adaptive design study can be the basis for requesting a Type C meeting. FDA's ability to address such requests for studies in early phases of drug development, however, may be limited and will depend on competing workload priorities and on the particulars of the drug and use under development. Innovative therapeutics for an area of unmet medical need are likely to garner more review attention than other products FDA believes do not fall into this category.

B. Late Stages of Drug Development

FDA has a more extensive role in assessing the design of studies that contribute to substantial evidence of effectiveness. FDA's review focus in later stages of drug development continues to include safety of study subjects, but also includes assuring that studies performed at this stage contain plans for assessment of safety and efficacy that will result in data of sufficient quality and quantity to inform a regulatory decision. Regulatory mechanisms for obtaining formal, substantive, feedback from FDA on design of the later stage trials and their place in the drug development program are well established (e.g., the End-of-Phase 2 (EOP2) meeting and Special Protocol Assessments (SPA)).

Depending on the preexisting breadth and depth of information regarding the drug, its specific use, and the nature of the adaptive features, an EOP2 meeting may be the appropriate place in development for initial discussion of an adaptive design A&WC study. However, if there is only limited knowledge of certain critical aspects of the drug's use before conducting the adaptive study, and the study is intended to obtain such knowledge using the study's adaptive features (particularly less well-understood methods), discussion with FDA earlier than usual is advisable (e.g., at a Type C or End-of-Phase 2A meeting). An early meeting for A&WC study protocols with complex adaptive features allows time to carefully consider the plan and to revise and reevaluate it as appropriate, without slowing the clinical development program. This early discussion should specifically address the adaptive methodology in general and the suitability of the selected approach to achieve the study's goals. This early, focused adaptive design discussion may not eliminate the value of a subsequent EOP2 meeting.

FDA's review of proposed A&WC studies in a drug development program includes considering whether the totality of the existing information combined with the expected information from the proposed studies will likely be adequate to enable a review of a marketing application for approval. This analysis is often enhanced by an EOP2 meeting that includes assessing the adequacy of plans for evaluating the drug's dose-response, treatment-regimen selection, choice of patient population, and other important aspects of the therapy's use.

It is important to recognize that use of less well-understood adaptive methods may limit FDA's ability to offer such an assessment. FDA may be unable to assess in advance whether the adaptively selected aspects of drug use (e.g., dose, regimen, population) will be sufficiently justified by the study results. As usual, FDA will review and comment to the extent possible on aspects of the drug's use that the sponsor considers well defined, as well as non-adaptive aspects of the study.

As previously discussed, FDA will generally not be involved in examining the interim data used for the adaptive decision-making and will not provide comments on the adaptive decisions while the study is ongoing. FDA's review and acceptance at the protocol design stage of the methodology for the adaptation process does not imply its advance concurrence that the adaptively selected choices will be the optimal choices. For example, if for feasibility of design, the adaptive selection of dose is based on one aspect of a drug's effect, but the optimal choice depends on the interplay between two aspects of drug effect, the data resulting from the study will be evaluated to judge whether adequate dose selection has been made.

C. Special Protocol Assessments

Special protocol assessments (SPA) entail timelines (45-day responses) and commitments that may not be best suited for adaptive design studies. The full review and assessment of a study using less well-understood adaptive design methods can be complex, will involve a multidisciplinary evaluation team, and might involve extended discussions among individuals within different FDA offices before reaching a conclusion.

If there has been little or no prior discussion between FDA and the study sponsor regarding the proposed study and its adaptive design features, other information requests following initial FDA evaluation are likely and full completion of study assessment within the SPA 45-day time frame is unlikely. Sponsors are therefore encouraged to have thorough discussions with FDA (as noted in section X.B above) regarding the study design and the study's place within the development program before considering submitting an SPA request.

Even when adequate advance discussion has occurred, the nature of a full protocol assessment of an adaptive design study may not be the same as for an SPA request for a conventional study, as one or more critical final decisions regarding study design are made after the study has started. FDA cannot realistically commit to accepting aspects of study design yet to be determined. Thus, although an adaptive design SPA request that had been preceded by adequate advance discussion, enabling a complete protocol review, the FDA response may have certain limitations that an SPA regarding a non-adaptive study would not require.

XI. DOCUMENTATION AND PRACTICES TO PROTECT STUDY BLINDING AND INFORMATION SHARING FOR ADAPTIVE DESIGNS

Protecting study blinding is important in all clinical trials, but in the case of an adaptive design study, where the design is modified after examination of unblinded interim data, protecting study blinding is particularly important to avoid the introduction of bias in the study conduct and to maintain confidence in the validity of the study's result.

In addition to the full documentation required for a study protocol (21 CFR 312.23(a)), there should be comprehensive and prospective, written standard operating procedures (SOPs) that define who will implement the interim analysis and adaptation plan, and all monitoring and related procedures for accomplishing the implementation, providing for the strict control of access to unblinded data (see the DMC guidance). SOPs for an adaptive design study with an unblinded interim analysis are likely to be more complex than SOPs for non-adaptive studies to ensure that there is no possibility of bias introduction.

This written documentation should include (1) identification of the personnel who will perform the interim analyses, and who will have access to the interim results, (2) how that access will be controlled and verified, and how the interim analyses will be performed, including how any potential irregularities in the data (e.g., withdrawals, missing values) will be managed, and (3) how adaptation decisions will be made. Other issues that should be addressed in these SOPs are (1) whether there are any foreseeable impediments to complying with the SOPs, (2) how compliance with the SOPs will be documented and monitored, and (3) what information, under what circumstances, is permitted to be passed from the DMC to the sponsor or investigators. It is likely that the measures defined by the SOPs will be related to the type of adaptation and the potential for impairing study integrity.

In general, a person or group that is independent of the personnel involved with conducting or potentially modifying (e.g., a steering committee) the study should be used for the review of an interim analysis of unblinded data and adaptive decision-making. This process should be based on the study management structure set in place by the study sponsor, steering committee, or other group responsible for the study, and in accordance with the well-specified adaptation plans.

This role could be assigned to an independent DMC when a DMC is established for other study monitoring purposes. DMCs typically will be provided certain kinds of information, of which some might be unblinded analyses, and procedures are usually in place to ensure that this information does not become available outside of the committee. Alternatively, a DMC might be delegated only the more standard roles (e.g., ongoing assessment of critical safety information) and a separate adaptation committee used to examine the interim analysis and make adaptation recommendations. In either case, the specific duties and procedures of the committees should be fully and prospectively documented.

The planned operating procedures should call for written minutes of all committee meetings that describe what was reviewed, discussed, and decided. Sponsors should plan for procedures to maintain these records in a secure manner with restricted access to enable post-study review of adherence to the prospective process. For the same purpose, the actual interim analysis results and a *snapshot* of the databases used for that interim analysis and adaptation decision should also be retained in a secure manner.

In recent years there has been greatly increased use of contract research organizations (clinical research organization) for many tasks previously performed by direct employees of the study sponsor. In particular, this has included assigning to clinical research organizations the task of performing the interim analysis and making study decisions based on the interim results.

Many clinical research organizations do not have long histories of carrying out these responsibilities. Study sponsors should have assurance that the personnel performing these roles have appropriate expertise, and that there are clear and adequate written SOPs to ensure compliance with the precautions needed to maintain study integrity. The clinical research organization should be able to maintain confidentiality of the information examined in the interim analysis and it should establish that it has the ability to do so.

A failure either to make the appropriate decisions as directed in the prospective SAP or to maintain confidentiality of the interim results might have an adverse impact on the interpretation of the study results. The processes established, as well as how they were performed, should be well documented in the final study report. The ability for FDA to verify compliance, potentially by on-site auditing, may be critical.

XII. EVALUATING AND REPORTING A COMPLETED STUDY

Sponsors often seek to communicate to FDA the results of a completed adaptive design study before undertaking a subsequent study within an investigational new drug application (IND). Marketing applications should always include study reports for completed studies.

To allow FDA to thoroughly review the results of adaptive design studies, complete and detailed documentation should be supplied in addition to the detailed information for the prospective FDA review of the protocol. All prospective plans and planning support information, detailed description of the study conduct in all aspects, and comprehensive analysis of results should be included in a marketing application submission. More limited information (e.g., reports without the database copies, less-detailed information on other aspects) may be sufficient for study summaries provided to FDA during the course of development to support ongoing discussions within the IND.

In addition to the guidance provided by the ICH E3 guidance regarding the format and content of a clinical study report, there are some unique features to reporting the conduct and analysis of an adaptive design study to FDA. Information submitted regarding the prospective plans should be complete. This information should include the study protocol and study procedure documents, including DMC or other committee charters. The submission should also include the supportive information that was developed to assist the sponsor in the prospective planning and FDA in the prospective review of the study. This information can include the rationale for using an adaptive design, the role of the study within the overall drug development program, and the simulations and other statistical evaluations performed prospectively. Submissions should include copies of published articles critical to assessing the methodology.

Complete information describing the study conduct should include the following:

- information on compliance with the planned adaptive process and procedures for maintaining study integrity,
- description of the processes and procedures actually carried out when there were any deviations from those planned,
- records of the deliberations and participants in the internal discussions by any committees (e.g., DMC meeting minutes, steering or executive committee meeting minutes) involved in the adaptive process,
- results of the interim analysis used for the adaptation decisions (including estimates of treatment effects, uncertainty of the estimates, and hypothesis tests at that time),
- assessment of adequacy of any firewalls established to limit dissemination of information.

Sponsors should consider using a diagrammatic display of the course of the study, illustrating the adaptive plan and the actual decisions made at each juncture. A copy of the study databases that were used for the interim analyses and adaptation decisions should be maintained in a data locked manner and also submitted. If there were multiple stages for adaptation with multiple interim analyses, each stage should be fully represented in the report, both as cumulative information and as information acquired during each stage separately. It is important to include all of this information for FDA evaluation of the study conduct, analysis, and interpretation.

The analysis of study final results should be complete and should adhere to the prospective analytic plan. Any deviations from the prospective plan should be detailed and discussed, and the sponsor should assess any potential bias in the results these deviations might have introduced. It may be important to include relevant exploratory analyses of the study data in this assessment.

Exploration of the study data should include examining the consistency of treatment effects and other relevant results between study stages. Statistical tests for differences in treatment-effect estimates between stages of the trial will generally have poor statistical power and are not by themselves a sufficient approach to this issue. Comparability between patients recruited before and after the adaptation can be examined, for instance, by baseline characteristics as well as clinical outcome. If these evaluations suggest a potential shift in population, outcome, or other parameters, more detailed evaluation will be warranted.

References

Chin, R., Lee, B.Y. Principles and Practice of Clinical Trial Medicine, Elsevier, St. Louis, 2008.

Committee for Medicinal Products for Human Use. Reflection Paper on Methodological Issues in Confirmatory Clinical Trials with Flexible Design and Analysis Plan, Draft. 2006. Accessed 15 July 2010.

EMA. Report on the EMEA-EFPIA Workshop on Adaptive Designs in Confirmatory Clinical Trials. http://www.ema.europa.eu/pdfs/conferenceflyers/report_adaptivedesigns.pdf. Accessed 15 July 2010.

FDA. Guidance for Industry: Adaptive Design Clinical Trials for Drugs and Biologics. 2010.

FDA. Guidance for the Use of Bayesian Statistics in Medical Device Clinical Trials. http://www.fda.gov/MedicalDevices/DeviceRegulationandGuidance/GuidanceDocuments/ucm071072.htm. Accessed 5 July 2010.

Sheiner, L.B. Learning versus confirming in clinical drug development. *Clin Pharmacol Ther*. 1997; 61:275–291.

Temple, B. Presentation at the Adaptive Designs Workshop, 2006.

2

Conventional Statistics

2.1 Basic Statistics

A comprehensive review of statistics is beyond the scope of this book. However, the science of adaptive clinical trials requires a good working knowledge of basic statistics, partly because the field is young and evolving, partly because much of the present literature on adaptive designs is statistical, and partly because adaptive designs require somewhat more sophisticated understanding of statistics than conventional trials. This chapter discusses conventional statistics and the next chapter discusses statistics specifically related to adaptive designs.

2.2 Statistical Schools

Statistics is an epistemological discipline. It is a way of taking a particular type of data—in this case, a large amount of numeric data—and drawing some conclusion about the world based on that data.

As you might imagine, there are many ways of taking a large set of numeric data and drawing conclusions. To date, statisticians have formulated three main ways of doing this: the frequentist method, Bayesian method, and likelihood method.

In traditional clinical studies, the frequentist method is almost always utilized. In fact, the frequentist school is so dominant today that most clinicians and even many statisticians are not familiar with the other statistical approaches. The frequentist approach is perfectly acceptable for traditional non-adaptive clinical trials but not for adaptive clinical trials. For adaptive clinical trials, the field will likely evolve toward a combination of three schools.

2.3 Frequentist Method

The current orthodox statistical approach in clinical research is the frequentist approach, based on Neyman, Pearson, and Fisher's pioneering works (Lehmann 1993).

The frequentist approach starts by defining a "null hypothesis," which, in clinical research, is usually a hypothesis that there are no differences in outcome between two treatment groups. The frequentist school analyzes the result of a study as follows. First, it asks, for any given clinical trial, what is the universe of potential possible results? For example, if there are three patients in each arm, and each patient can be a responder or a nonresponder, then there are $2 \times 2 \times 2$ possible results in each arm. There can be anywhere from zero to three responders in each arm, with one or two responders being most likely. If there are two arms, then there are 8×8 possible results, of which there are zero to three responders in one arm and zero to three responders in the other arm.

Second, it takes the results of a study and compares it against the universe of all potential results that could have been seen if the null hypothesis were true. If it is highly unlikely that the result would have been seen by chance if the null hypothesis were true, then the null hypothesis is rejected and the conclusion is that there are differences in the two treatment groups. For example, if there are two responders in each arm, then there are many possible permutations that could have resulted in two responders, so that is not an unlikely result. If there are three responders in one arm and zero in the other, then there is only one permutation that could have resulted in that outcome, out of 64 possible permutations, so that is not likely.

This likelihood is based on the p value, which is based on how extreme the study results are compared to the distribution of all possible results. The p value is a numeric representation of how unlikely the results are. If the p value is very small the results are not likely due to chance and the null hypothesis is rejected. If the p value is not small enough, the null hypothesis is not rejected.

The frequentist approach is relatively simple, robust, and does not require knowledge of prior probabilities. The frequentist method has the major advantage that no external information is required to interpret a study. That is, the analysis can be performed purely based on the data from a study and that data only. Therefore, it is the most common statistical method used in clinical research. There are significant downsides to this approach, though. One downside is that the p values only tell you whether there is a difference or not, not how great the difference is. The p value in and of itself does not give an indication of how large the difference is between the two groups. Clinical trialists have started relying on confidence intervals to overcome this limitation because confidence intervals provide an estimate of how large the difference is between the arms of the study.

Another disadvantage, especially where adaptive clinical trials are concerned, is that multiple comparisons are disallowed and that multiple looks at the data (for example, via interim analysis) can have a significant impact on the ultimate power of the study. In other words, one study can normally answer only one question, and multiple looks at the data are not easily performed. This is obviously a problem for adaptive designs that rely on multiple looks at the data.

In addition, the frequentist approach is nonintuitive to many people. For example, it is often difficult to understand the notion of "preassigning alpha." This notion is the rule that the primary endpoint of a study must be declared in advance. For example, let's say that a study shows a difference between treated and untreated group that yields a nominal p value of 0.0001. In this case, if the endpoint had been prespecified as the primary endpoint in advance, the study is positive. But if another endpoint had been declared as the primary endpoint, the exact same results would be considered to demonstrate a lack of efficacy.

Also, the p value from a study is defined not as the probability that the results are by chance. A p value of 0.01 does not mean that there is 1% chance that the positive results are spurious. Instead, it is supposed to represent what results could have been observed even if the events were actually not observed. It's based on the universe of all potential outcomes. For example, let's say there is a study that terminates after 100 deaths. Even with the exact same number of patients and deaths, the p value would depend on the reason for the study termination. If the study were terminated because the number of events had been reached, the p value would be different than if it were terminated because the follow-up period was complete. This is a confusing concept to grasp.

The need to declare the endpoint in advance is analogous the following example of a bet on free throws. If you were betting a friend on whether he would make at least one free throw, you would have different odds if he was allowed to try once or ten times. If he was a 50% free throw shooter, the odds would be 1:1 for a single try and about 1,000:1 for ten attempts. In the first instance, if would be a fair bet to wager $1 vs. $1. If he was to have ten attempts to get at least one free throw, a fair bet would be 1 cent vs. $10. Even if he made the free throw on the first try, if the agreement was that he would have up to ten attempts, he would not be allowed to claim 1:1 odds in retrospect and try to collect $1 instead of 1 cent.

Some of the confusion flows from an accident of history. It should be noted that though modern frequentist statistics is based on Neyman-Pearson and Fisher's work, it is a somewhat unnatural amalgamation of the two schools (Lehmann 1993). Neyman-Pearson's statistics do not make use of p values but rather alpha and Type I and II errors, whereas Fisher's relies on p values and not on Type I or II errors. Alpha and p values are not the same, although they are generally treated as such. The traditional frequentist statistics used today is a somewhat incongruent mix of the two schools.

2.4 Bayesian Method

Bayesian school's approach to statistical analysis is the one closest to everyday logic that most people use in life. It asks the question, "Given what we know about the situation, and given the additional data from the study, how does it change our view of reality?" It takes prior probabilities (e.g., we believe that there is 70% chance that the drug works) and adds additional data to the probability to arrive at a posterior probability (e.g., we now believe there is 90% chance that the drug works). It has several major advantages, including intuitiveness, the ability to take multiple looks at data from a study, and finer gradations or richer sets of conclusions.

Its major drawback is the difficulty of assigning prior probabilities, or the starting set of beliefs. This limitation is particularly acute in traditional clinical trials, because the reason for performing clinical trials is often that there is no reliable prior probability regarding the efficacy of a drug or an intervention.

Bayesian methods are also prone to one of the most important frequentist shortcomings. Both methods can suffer from sampling to a foregone conclusion. If you are allowed to take multiple looks at the data and continue sampling as long as the data do not support your viewpoint but are allowed to stop if and when the data turn in your favor, neither frequentist nor Bayesian methodologies will protect you from potentially spurious positive results.

2.5 Likelihood Method

Likelihood analysis assigns relative likelihood between two or more competing interpretations of the data, based on the results of the study. It asks the question, "If we had to pick between view A of reality and view B of reality, which would we pick?" It does not require prior probability, nor is it hobbled by limitations on multiple comparisons.

However, its major limitation is that the choice of alternative hypothesis has a critical effect on the usefulness of the conclusions, and it does not speak to the relationship between the proposed hypothesis and the unarticulated alternate hypotheses. It speaks to the comparative likelihood of the alternate stated hypothesis but does not speak to the likelihood vs. unlikelihood of either hypothesis. In other words, it doesn't speak to "What about C?" or "Is either A or B or both plausible or is one just less implausible than the other?"

2.6 Other Schools

There are multiple other schools of analysis, including some incipient work on pattern-matching causation analysis, which is more intuitive than any of the above methods, but they are underdeveloped at present.

2.7 Descriptive Statistics

Broadly speaking, there are several different types of statistical analysis. The simplest is descriptive statistics. This type is exactly as it sounds: you take the data and describe it. Usually, the most useful technique is to take a lot of data points and distill the data into a handful of "summary statistics" that tell you what the data look like. For example, you might take height measurements from 1,000 people and summarize them with mean height and standard deviation. That way, you or someone else could look at two summary statistics and get a sense of what the height data look like, instead of looking at 1,000 data points individually.

2.8 Inferential Statistics

Often, however, there are things that you want to know about but that are impractical to measure, such as the height of everyone in the United States. Other things may be impossible to measure, such as the number of additional days of life that drug X adds to all past, present, and future breast cancer patients who have received or will receive the drug. In such cases, you take a subset of the data, say 1,000 random U.S. citizens, and extrapolate from that subset what the population at large might look like. This subset of the data is called a *sample*. The entire population from which the subset is drawn is called the *population*. The process of extrapolating the results of the analysis of the sample to the population at large is called *inferential statistics*.

Inferential statistics is at the heart of clinical research. This is in contrast to most other scientific fields, which are deterministic or deductive. In sciences such as physics, an experiment that produces a predicted result can be considered to validate the hypothesis. Two hydrogens bonded to an oxygen is always water, 2×10 is always 20, and e is always equal to mc^2. In many other scientific disciplines, once the assumptions and the scientific principles are known, the conclusion is always calculable. This is because the results are often fully determined—in other words, a unique set of causes exists for a unique set of results. For example, if matter is converted into energy, and the resultant amount of energy is known, then the amount of starting matter must be of a certain value.

In clinical trials, this is not the case. Clinical trials are stochastic, or probability based. It is not possible in stochastic science to prove or disprove something definitively; it is only possible to infer that something is probable/plausible/likely or not because the results can vary even for the same set of causes.

To make things even more counterintuitive, for most clinical trials, you cannot even directly establish that an outcome is likely the result of some precedent event. You can only establish that an outcome is not likely the result of the opposite precedent event. For example, you conclude that a drug is likely to improve an outcome by demonstrating that it is unlikely that there is no difference in outcome between the treated and the untreated group.

This is because of the variability in clinical course. A completely ineffective intervention could, purely by chance, yield clinical trial results that make it appear that the intervention is effective and vice versa. In other words, in clinical trials, 2 × 10 is usually 20 but could sometimes be 40, and 4 × 10 is usually 40 but could sometimes be 20. And an intervention that decreases blood pressure by 10 mmHg would decrease blood pressure by 10 mmHg in clinical trials on average if an infinite number of trials were run, but for any given trial, it could decrease it by 9 mmHg or 15 mmHg or even increase it.

In addition, because clinical trials are stochastic, and because of the variability inherent in medicine, clinical trials results are overdetermined (Figure 2.1). There is more than one set of circumstances that can lead to similar clinical trial results. Therefore, it is not sufficient to show merely that an outcome is a reasonable consequence of an intervention, because that

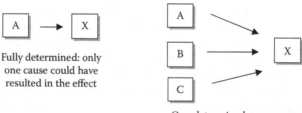

Determinism

Fully determined: only one cause could have resulted in the effect

Overdetermined: many causes could have resulted in the effect

IGURE 2.1
Determinism.

does not exclude the possibility that the same outcome is a reasonable consequence of another factor or even random chance.

For example, if one small trial shows that an intervention decreases blood pressure by 10 mmHg, it does not necessarily prove that the drug decreases blood pressure by that much. Similarly, it is not enough to show that an active arm with 10% mortality and a placebo arm with 20% is consistent with the drug being active. If there is enough variability in the population, the same result could also be consistent with the drug not being active. A 10 mmHg drop in blood pressure could be from a placebo effect. Or the drug might really decrease blood pressure by 5 mmHg or actually increase it, but the placebo effect is overwhelming the drug effect.

In the real world, especially in the biological world, where the variables are infinite, no two things are exactly the same. There is variability in height, weight, speed, and other features of biological phenomenon. In pragmatic terms, even measurement performed in deterministic science has variability. The difference is that the true value is still deterministic, and the more accurate the measurement, the better the prediction of outcome. In biological realms, no matter how accurate the measurement, there is still variability that persists. Measuring blood pressure to 0.01 mmHg will not strengthen the conclusions about whether the drug works.

Because of the variability, there is always a distribution of values for any given population.

Because there is variability, it is impossible to know exactly what the results will be for an intervention with a drug, etc. However, by knowing the distribution and the variability, we can make predictions about what is likely to occur. For example, we can say that a drug will lower the blood pressure an average of 5 mmHg, and we can say what the standard deviation is.

2.9 Comparative Statistics

Comparative statistics compares two or more groups. Often, the question of interest in a clinical trial concerns comparing two or more groups. For example, the most common question of interest in clinical research is "Did a group that received the drug fare better than the group that did not?" In these cases, you can take a sample of patients who received the drug and a sample of patients who did not and compare the two. Based on the differences between the two samples, you can infer what the differences are between the entire populations. This type of analysis—taking people who have received the drug and those who have not and comparing the two—is a very common type of analysis.

2.10 Hypothesis Testing

When you compare two groups of patients who have been exposed to different therapies, one potential issue is bias. There might be a reason that one group received one therapy and the other another therapy. That reason might be the cause of the outcome difference rather than the treatments. For example, perhaps one group received different therapy because that group was sicker.

The only sure way—and the best way—of eliminating the above type of bias is to avoid looking at the past and look forward instead. When you analyze data that have been collected about what has already happened, that is called a *retrospective study*. When you design the study first and then collect data on future events, that is called a *prospective study*.

Retrospective studies can only be observational. *Observational* means that you collect data about what occurred but do not try to change what happens. You're like an anthropologist, not interfering in local culture.

Prospective studies can be observational or interventional. *Interventional* means that you intervene in how a patient is treated. Most commonly, you decide who will get the drug and who will get a placebo. If you assign the treatment to the patients impartially, you will eliminate much of the bias we have been talking about. Assigning the treatment randomly, or by randomization, is the best, although not the only, way of assigning treatment impartially. If the randomization is performed properly, the two samples will be similar in every way except for the treatment or lack of treatment. This will make it easier to ascribe any differences in outcome to the difference in treatment assignment.

The traditional statistical technique used to establish causation is called *hypothesis testing*.

2.11 Null Hypothesis and Standard of Proof in Clinical Trials

A priori, the most useful hypothesis to test in clinical trials would seem to be a hypothesis that posits something, such as "This intervention increases survival by 10%" or "This intervention reduces blood pressure by 10 mmHg." However, clinical trials use a null hypothesis such as "This intervention has no effect." This is a peculiarity that is fundamental to the design and science of clinical trials.

Because it is not possible to prove that an intervention caused the outcome, one must show that a lack of intervention (probably) did not cause the outcome. In order to draw a conclusion that the result was due to an intervention, one must show that it is unlikely that it was not due to intervention.

This is why the null hypothesis is usually stated in the form, "There is no difference between the active and the control groups."

This approach of establishing cause and effect by disproving the null hypothesis has inherent limitations. The conventional p value of 0.05 is arbitrary. The outcome is dichotomous and does not yield information such as the magnitude of the effect difference or the point estimate of the effect. A trial therefore could be positive without being great enough in magnitude to be of clinical significance. It does not yield information about subgroups. It is a dichotomous answer to a multifaceted question. Nonetheless, it is the best method devised to date to investigate the causal relationship between clinical intervention and clinical outcome.

An Analogy

A person is visiting the United States but does not speak or read English. He decides to go for a walk from his hotel and not wanting get lost, writes down the name of the street on a piece of paper. Later, he loses his way as he thought he might. Fortunately, he has his piece of paper with him, and he stops a stranger to ask for help. He shows the stranger his paper, and on it is written, "One Way."

Obviously, the only way for this person to make sure that what he writes down doesn't say "One Way" or "Stop" or other similar signs would be to check other streets and rule out that he is not writing down something that is not a street name. Clinical research is similar in that it is not sufficient to determine that a result is consistent with a hypothesis. It is necessary to demonstrate that other hypotheses are inconsistent.

2.12 Example of Inference and Hypothesis Testing

So how exactly does inference work? We will start with an example. Let's say your friend has a garden that has roses and lilies. Let's say that they grew from seeds that were sown and you wanted to figure out whether

- The seeds were sown together at the same time from a mixed seed bag of "Special Rose and Lily Seed Mix" (hypothesis 1).
- They were sown separately, once from "Rupert's Red Rose Seeds" and "Lovely Lily Seeds" (hypothesis 2).

As an analogy, these two hypotheses are analogous to the following hypotheses often used in clinical trials:

- The drug had no effect on outcome. The results seen from the active and the placebo groups are the same (null hypothesis).
- The drug changed the outcome. The results seen from the active group are different from the results seen from the placebo group (reject null hypothesis).

Looking at Figures 2.2 and 2.3, which do you think is compatible with hypotheses 1 and 2?

Of course, Figure 2.2 is more compatible with the hypothesis that they were sown together.

However, you cannot ever say for sure that they were sown together because there are other possible ways they could have ended up growing that way. For example, maybe rose seeds were sown one day and the lily seeds the next day but just in the same place. Or maybe two people walking

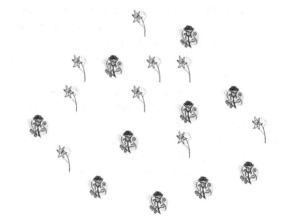

FIGURE 2.2
Roses and lilies.

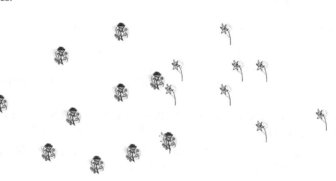

FIGURE 2.3
Roses and lilies.

side by side sowed them, one person sowing the roses, one person sowing the lilies.

On the other hand, it is possible to be pretty sure that they were not sown together if the flowers were growing in a pattern like the one you see in Figure 2.3. If would be pretty unlikely that you would have a distribution that is so different if they were sown from a mix of seeds from the same bag.

This illustrates a point that, in statistics, it is almost impossible to prove that two things are equal—just as it is impossible to definitively say that roses and lilies were sown together in Figure 2.2. It is possible, however, to say that two things are not equal, just as we can say about the roses and lilies in Figure 2.3 were not sown together.

Now, what is it about the second picture that makes you say that the seeds were probably not sown together? It is probably because the clustering of the roses in one place and the lilies in the other. This conclusion is intuitive to most people.

2.13 Statistical Tests and Choice of Statistical Test

Of course, intuition alone is not a sufficient way of hypothesis testing. Statistics formalizes this intuition into mathematical numbers. Much of frequentist statistics is based on taking the distribution of values—in this case, the distribution of the flower locations—and converting that information into some sort of a number. This number is called a *test variable* and is essentially a measure of how weird or unexpected the distribution is, compared to what might have been expected. If it is very weird, then the original hypothesis is rejected.

Essentially, you take the observed distribution, quantify it in some way (such as some formula based on mean value and standard deviation from each treatment group), and divide it by the expected distribution (such as some formula based on mean value and standard error from both treatment groups combined). You would get the following after you do this:

$$\frac{\text{Values that are observed}}{\text{Values that are expected}}$$

If this ratio (test variable) is very different from 1, that would make it likely that the assumption that two treatment groups are the same (the null hypothesis) is wrong.

Now, how do you know how weird the test variable is, and when is it weird enough to say that the results do not match up with the null hypothesis? Let's address the second part of that question first. By convention, if the likelihood of obtaining the results you obtained is less than 5%, then we say that the results are statistically significant. This is pure convention—most researchers have just agreed to the 5%, but it is completely arbitrary. The likelihood of obtaining the results you obtained is expressed as a p value. We will discuss p values later in this chapter.

Now, how do you obtain the p value? Most people would say, "You take the test variable and you look up the p value in a table" or "You use the computer program." This is true, but it is important to understand where those tables come from.

2.14 Examples of Statistical Tests

Depending on the type of statistical test you are using (t test, chi-square test, etc.), the tables are different, but they are derived in a similar way. We will take as an example the roll of two dice. We want to know whether these dice are loaded or fair. We know that if the dice are fair, there is an equal chance that we will get each one of the following combinations:

	1	2	3	4	5	6
1	1 + 1	1 + 2	1 + 3	1 + 4	1 + 5	1 + 6
2	2 + 1	2 + 2	2 + 3	2 + 4	2 + 5	2 + 6
3	3 + 1	3 + 2	3 + 3	3 + 4	3 + 5	3 + 6
4	4 + 1	4 + 2	4 + 3	4 + 4	4 + 5	4 + 6
5	5 + 1	5 + 2	5 + 3	5 + 4	5 + 5	5 + 6
6	6 + 1	6 + 2	6 + 3	6 + 4	6 + 5	6 + 6

There are thirty-six possible combinations. The sum of the two dice ranges from two to twelve. If you plotted the sums you would get the distribution seen in Figure 2.4.

Now, this graph can be expressed in terms of the percentage of the time that you will see the sum rather than the frequency in Figure 2.4(B).

Now you can draw up a table that expresses the likelihood of getting a particular sum or more extreme, as shown in Table 2.1.

So, for example, you roll the dice and they come up a 1 and a 2. You want to know how likely it is that you would arrive at such a low number (sum of three or less), so you look it up and find that it is 8% likely you would get a three or less, which is equivalent to a p value of 0.08.

Most statistical test tables are constructed in a similar way—you list out all of the possible combinations and figure out how often you see a particularly extreme event. When you cannot list out all of the possible combinations,

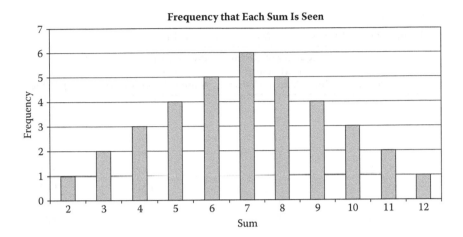

FIGURE 2.4A
Distribution of dice sums.

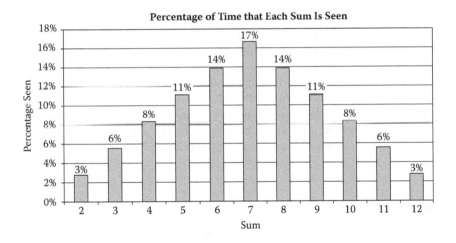

FIGURE 2.4B
Result of dice sums by frequency.

you can use a mathematical formula, making some assumptions about how the values are distributed.

Depending on the type of data, how many arms there are that you are comparing, and whether you are comparing sets of data from the same group of individuals or only one piece of data from each person, there are various types of tests. For continuous variables with two sets of data, as an example, the most common test is the *t* test. This is a test that compares the mean and the standard deviation between the two groups and determines whether the samples look like they came from the same population or different

TABLE 2.1

Likelihood of Rolling Value or More Extreme Value

Sum	Frequency	Frequency of Getting as Extreme or More Extreme Values	Probability of Observing as Extreme or More Extreme Values (%)	p Value
2	1	1	3	0.03
3	2	3	8	0.08
4	3	6	17	0.17
5	4	10	28	0.28
6	5	15	42	0.42
7	6	36	100	1.00
8	5	15	42	0.42
9	4	10	28	0.28
10	3	6	17	0.17
11	2	3	8	0.08
12	1	1	3	0.03

populations. If the standard deviation is high and the means are similar, then it is likely that they came from the same population; if the reverse is true, then it is not likely.

For a dichotomous variable, the chi-square test is often used. In this test, the boxes of a distribution are examined to see how likely it is that the squares would have been populated as if it was by chance. For small samples, Fisher's exact test is preferred, and for very large samples, the z-test can be used. A description of these tests is summarized in Table 2.2.

2.15 Fundamental Statistical Assumptions

2.15.1 Background

As mentioned previously, all statistical procedures and tests make certain assumptions. All of the statistical techniques that are used in clinical research to make comparisons between groups have to make an assumption regarding how the values are distributed. In fact, it is not possible to draw any conclusions from comparisons without making an assumption about the distribution because, in effect, the question that is asked during the comparisons is "Does this distribution of values look right?" or, more specifically, "Does this distribution of values look the like what we expected?" Many times the assumption is that the distribution is normal. The statistical

TABLE 2.2

Types of Statistical Tests

Measurement Type	Continuous, Parametric	Nominal/ Ordinal/ Nonparametric	Dichotomous (Two Possible Outcomes)	Survival (Time to Event)
Describe one group	Mean, standard deviation	Median, percentiles	Proportion	Kaplan-Meier survival curve, Median survival
Compare one group to a hypothetical value	One-sample *t* test	Wilcoxon test	Chi-square or binominal test	
Compare two unpaired groups	Unpaired *t* test	Mann-Whitney	Fisher's or chi-square	Log-rank or Mantel-Haenszel
Compare two paired groups	Paired *t* test	Wilcoxon	McNemar's	Conditional proportional hazards regression
Compare three or more unmatched groups	One-way analysis of variance	Kruskal-Wallis	Chi-square	Cox proportional hazards regression
Compare three or more matched groups	Repeated-measures analysis of variance	Friedman	Cochrane's *Q*	Conditional proportional hazards regression
Quantify relationship between two variables	Pearson's correlation	Spearman correlation	Contingency coefficients	
Predict value from another variable	Linear (or nonlinear) regression	Nonparametric regression	Simple logistic regression	Cox proportional hazards regression
Predict values from several measured or binominal variables	Multiple linear (or nonlinear) regression		Multiple logistic regression	Cox proportional hazards regression

Source: This table is derived from Motulsky, H., *Intuitive Statistics*, Oxford Press, 1995.

techniques that make this assumption of normal distribution are referred to as *parametric tests*.

In many cases, slight violations of the assumptions will not have a material effect on the results. However, in some cases they can. Therefore, it is important for the clinician, not just the statistician, to be aware of the assumptions. It is the clinician's responsibility to inform the statistician if the assumptions are violated. Obviously, it is critical to provide this input to the statistician, because if one or more of the assumptions are violated, the statistical test

TABLE 2.3

Types of Statistical Tests

Measurement Type	Single Center	Multicenter or Strata	Model Based
Dichotomous	Fisher's exact Chi-square	Mantel–Haenszel	Logistic regression
Nominal	Chi-square	Extended Mantel–Haenszel	Log-linear model
Ordinal or discrete counts	Rank-sum	Extended Mantel–Haenszel	Proportional odds model
Time to event	Log rank	Extended Mantel–Haenszel (log rank) for survival data	Proportional hazards
Continuous	Rank-sum *t* Test	Van Elteren	Multiple linear regression and analysis of covariance

would be inappropriate. One example would be a disease that has a nonlinear progression. Another example would be the fact that the standard treatment paradigm typically changes once a patient reaches a certain stage of disease. Statisticians, without the clinician's help, cannot know these types of facts. It is critical to discuss these factors with the statistician in advance of the study.

It is extremely important to work closely with the statistician when designing endpoints because the clinician must supply the critical information (such as if hazards are expected to cross) in order to not only select the appropriate analysis but to select the appropriate parameters to put into the analysis.

2.15.2 Parametric Assumption

The parametric assumption is one of the most common and most important assumptions used in many of the statistical procedures for clinical research.

Most things that we measure in nature have a "normal" or "Gaussian" distribution. That means that if the values are graphed, the result is a characteristic shape that looks a bit like a bell (bell-shaped curve). This is due to a mathematical property known as the *central limit theorem*, which notes that any event that is driven by a number of independent random influences tends to end up as a normal distribution. Also, as per the theorem, when multiple samples are obtained from any type of observation, the distribution of the samples tends to be normal. This is important because an analysis of samples derived even from a nonnormal population can be normal.

Also, it may be that the human mind categorizes and measures things in nature such that most things assume a normal distribution. For example, we perceive and measure length in inches or feet in a linear manner as opposed to inches squared or inverse of inches. This results in a normal distribution of height in the human population. It would not be a normal curve if we measured people's height on a logarithmic scale.

Normal distribution, bell-shaped curve, and *Gaussian distribution* all mean the same thing, and the assumption of this shape is the parametric assumption.

Normal distribution has one peak, is shaped like a bell, and is symmetrical; 68% of the values lie within one standard deviation of the mean, 95% within two standard deviations, and 99.7% within three standard deviations.

If a distribution is not normal, it can usually be mathematically transformed to a normal distribution.

In general, most biological phenomena take on a normal distribution, and when the study consists of multiple samples of something, the distribution is close to normal. However, for some measurements, and for small sample sizes, parametric tests are not appropriate. For example, blood pressure is normally distributed, but blood pressure in an intensive care unit or in a catheterization lab may not be.

Most statistical tests also assume that the variances in the groups being compared are similar.

2.15.3 Continuity and Linearity Assumptions

One common assumption in clinical research is that measurements are continuous and linear. For example, the difference between blood pressure of 100 and 110 is assumed to be similar in clinical value as the difference between 120 and 130. That's why clinicians accept statements such as, "This blood pressure drug decreases mean blood pressure by 6 mmHg."

However, biological phenomena are never truly continuous, although in practice they usually approximate it and are usually treated as such. For example, the difference between blood pressure of 60 and 90 is not similar in significance as the difference between 120 and 150. It is important to make the statistician aware of any nonlinearity in the values. For example, patients who present with a myocardial infarction and a very low or very high blood pressure have poor prognosis—this is a U-shaped curve.

2.15.4 Constant Hazard Ratio Assumptions

For survival analysis, one common assumption is that the risk of an event is constant over time. This assumption is particularly important with a Cox proportional hazards model, because it is particularly sensitive to it. If the survival curves cross or converge at the end, or even if the relative rates change, this assumption is violated.

2.15.5 Independent and Random Sampling

Another assumption that is important to statistical tests but is rarely well fulfilled in clinical research is the assumption that patients are drawn at random from the entire pool of patients with the disease. In actual studies, however, patient recruitment is not random, and this almost always introduces some bias into the study.

2.15.6 Independence of Events

Often, there is an assumption that outcomes are independent. For example, it is assumed that if a patient has a myocardial infarction, it will not cause other patients in the group to have a myocardial infarction. In some cases, this might not be the case. For example, in diseases where there is a strong subjective component in the endpoints or measurement instruments such as depression, pain, or ischemic bowel disease, patients visiting the site at the same time might talk with one another and influence each other. Or, as another example, one episode of atrial fibrillation might make it more likely that the patient will have another episode.

References

Lehmann, E. L. 1993. Neyman-Pearson. Theories of Testing Hypothesis. *J Am. Stat. Assc.* 88:1242–1249.
Motulsky, H. 1995. *Intuitive Statistics.* Oxford University Press.

3

Statistics Used in Adaptive Clinical Trials[*]

3.1 Introduction

Either frequentist or Bayesian analysis can be used for adaptive trials. Statistical techniques using both schools have also been developed. However, the frequentist or an adaptation of the frequentist approach has been developed much more thoroughly because the dominant paradigm in clinical trials is the frequentist method. Therefore, the frequentist approach is much more typical than the Bayesian approach even for adaptive clinical trials, even though the Bayesian approach is much more naturally suited for adaptive designs. Because most statistical techniques in the adaptive clinical trial literature are based on a frequentist approach, this chapter will focus mostly on them.

3.2 Preserving the Alpha

Using a frequentist approach, the alpha of 0.05 must be preserved in order to allow determination that the study is positive. If the p value is not less than 0.05, a conclusion of a causal relationship between the intervention and outcome cannot be drawn.

Adaptive clinical trials depend on conducting multiple analyses (or "looks") of the data during the course of the trial. Each analysis must be conducted in a meticulous fashion, with prespecification of how and what analysis will be done and what decision will be taken, as well as how much of the 0.05 alpha will be "spent." The total amount of alpha that is spent in the course of the study must not exceed 0.05, and the alpha must be carefully accounted for. Otherwise, there is Type I error inflation. That means that the likelihood of a spuriously positive study increases because multiple looks at the data and multiple chances for a study to be positive make the false-positive rate

---

[*] Sections 3.1–3.7 and 3.11 are based on Chin and Lee, 2008, with permission.

higher than 5%. Type I error inflation typically occurs when the criteriob of 0.05 is used over and over again without accounting for the fact that previous analyses have been performed. Because there is 5% chance that the analysis will be positive purely by chance every time it is conducted, given enough looks, one of the analyses will reach a p value of 0.05 or less.

Most modern advances in the statistics of adaptive trial design therefore focus on preserving the alpha through each and every look at the data. Preserving the alpha refers to the process of making sure that each time a decision is made regarding the trial, the likelihood of Type I error does not increase. This is typically done by carefully calculating and keeping track of exactly how much alpha has been spent. Alpha is spent each time unblinded results are used to make a decision.

The amount that is spent is dependent on how extreme the value of the outcome has to be before it influences the decision. Extreme values require less alpha to be spent. For example, let's say an interim analysis is performed. If it is determined in advance that the study will be stopped if the p value is less than 0.001, less alpha will be spent than if the criterion for stopping the study is set at a p value of less than 0.01. The amount of alpha spent is roughly equivalent to the p value used as the criterion for stopping the study or otherwise influencing the study.

However, the methodology of adding up the allocations is more complicated than simple addition. There are several different ways of accounting for the amount of alpha spent, described in detail in Section 3.6. Some of the alpha spending overlaps across the different analyses, so compensation for alpha that has already been allocated is sometimes necessary.

3.3 What Is Alpha?

Alpha refers to the significance level for a study. The significance level is the threshold number that the p value calculated for the prespecified primary endpoint must meet in order for the study to be considered positive. Typically, alpha is set at 5%, which means that the p value must be less than 0.05 in order for the study to be considered statistically significant. In some cases, alpha may be set at different levels, such as 0.025 or 0.10. As an illustration, the U.S. Food and Drug Administration (FDA) requires that the alpha be set at 0.00125 (0.05×0.05 divided by 2) if a sponsor is relying on a single pivotal study rather than two pivotal studies each with alpha of 0.05 or less.

Often, alpha is confused with probability of Type I error, even in statistical textbooks. Type I error, if you recall, is the mistake of rejecting the null hypothesis when it is actually true; for example, deciding that a treatment is better than placebo when it actually is not. Alpha and Type I error boundaries are both conventionally set at 0.05 or less in clinical trials. Functionally, they are used interchangeably but the two are distinct concepts. Type I (and Type II) errors were invented by Pearson and Neyman and refer to the probability of drawing wrong conclusions (Lehmann 1993). Alpha was invented by Fisher and refers to the likelihood that the result seen is due to chance rather than due to a real difference (Lehmann 1993). Meeting the alpha boundary leads to results in the study being *statistically significant*.

It is also important not to confuse *nominal p* values with *p* values. *p* Values can be calculated for any comparison, but unless they are for the prespecified primary endpoint they are nominal *p* values. There is only one *p* value for any study: the *p* value calculated for the primary endpoint. All others are nominal *p* values that cannot lead to causal conclusions. For example, let's say that a study is conducted in hypertension patients. The primary endpoint is the change in systolic pressure at 6 weeks. The *p* value is calculated for the primary endpoint and it is 0.11. The study does not meet statistical significance. The sponsor decides to calculate the nominal *p* value for change in systolic pressure at 4 weeks (which was not prespecified in the protocol), which may be 0.01, but that would not meet statistical significance because the primary endpoint was missed.

It is a common mistake to perform multiple comparisons, and multiple *ad hoc* analyses, and to assume a relationship just because the nominal *p* value is less than 0.05 when in reality the correlation is by chance. This type of misinterpretation is particularly common when the spurious relationship makes intuitive sense due to pathophysiology. This is because the human tendency is to look for causality and to believe the causality if it makes sense.

Please remember that there can be only one primary endpoint (except in instances where hierarchical testing is used or the alpha is divided), and it must be declared in advance. You cannot take a host of endpoints at the end of a study, perform statistical tests on them, and select the one that looks the best. This prohibition sounds simple but, in practice, many people fail to follow it. Here is a typical example:

A study in chronic obstructive pulmonary disease (COPD) patients is performed, with hospitalizations as the primary endpoint. Unfortunately, clinical practice guidelines for COPD change in the middle of the study, and the criteria for admission to the hospital are made more strict. As a result, the number of hospitalizations is much lower than expected. The study therefore becomes underpowered, and though there is 25% reduction in hospitalization, the *p* value is 0.08. However, it turns out that the mortality in the treated group is markedly lower than the placebo group, with 70% reduction in the mortality rate and a *p* value of 0.002. Not only that, but in the patients who received the full course of the drug, the reduction in mortality is 90% and the *p* value is 0.00001!

There is only one acceptable interpretation of the above example: the study results are negative, and there is no evidence that the drug has any beneficial effect. The issue is that if you look hard enough, you can find endpoints with

p values of 0.05 or less in any failed study. You cannot scrounge for a favorable endpoint and thereby rescue a failed study. The p value has meaning only for the primary endpoint. Unfortunately, it would not be uncommon for the investigator with results like the above to declare that the drug has an effect.

3.4 Misconception about p Values

The other common misconception about p values is that the smaller the p value, the greater the magnitude of the treatment effect. This is erroneous. Here is an example:

> Two companies are neck and neck in racing to develop a therapy for a congenital storage disease. Their drugs are nearly identical, but when the two companies announce their Phase II results nearly simultaneously, the results appear quite different.

- The first company announces a successful study with a $p = 0.0001$.
- The second announces a successful study with $p = 0.04$.

What happened? Did the second company make a mistake in their trial design? Is the first company's drug more likely to work?

No, the drugs worked similarly and to a similar magnitude in the two studies. However, the first company's study had 300 patients and the second company's had 80. p Values reflect two things: how well the drug works and how large the sample size is.

Impressive p values do not necessarily mean that a drug works better, if the studies are not equivalent in design and size.

In other words, smaller p values can come from either the drug working very well or from having a large number of patients in the study. You should not confuse the two.

Finally, remember when not to rely on p values. It is appropriate to require a p value of less than 0.05 when the objective is to establish efficacy for a new therapy. It is not appropriate to require a p value of 0.05 when assessing safety signals. The bar for safety should be much lower. Even a p value of 0.5 may be meaningful if the consequences of risk are great enough.

For example, if you are studying a drug for asthma, and there is an imbalance in the rate of heart attacks, you should take the signal very seriously even if the p value is not even close to 0.05. You are weighing a non-life-saving benefit against a life-threatening adverse event. The two are not equivalent. Waiting until the p value becomes significant may result in tremendous, irreparable harm being done. You would not wait until there was

95% chance of a fire before taking out fire insurance; nor should you wait until you are 95% sure there is a safety issue before taking action.

3.5 Splitting the Alpha

Even before modern adaptive clinical trials were developed, there were instances where alpha had to be allocated or divided. One common instance was if more than one primary endpoint was desired. For example, if a study were being performed in diabetes, one primary endpoint might be hemoglobin A1C and another endpoint might be glucose levels. Each endpoint could be tested for significance at a 0.025 level. In this case alpha of 0.05 has been divided equally into two 0.025 tests.

You can split the alpha across different endpoints unequally as well. For example, even if you only have two arms (active and placebo groups), you might assign an alpha of 0.04 for one endpoint such as survival and 0.01 for another endpoint such as reduction in hospitalization.

Another instance where this is necessary is in the case of multiple comparisons: looking at the same endpoint across many groups. Similar to a case with multiple endpoints, the alpha is divided or split. Alpha splitting means that you take 0.05 and allocate it across several different primary patient groups. For example, a study might be performed in myocardial infarction patients. One primary endpoint might be survival in all enrolled patients. Another primary endpoint might be survival in only patients with anterior myocardial infarctions. Each endpoint could be tested for significance at a 0.025 level.

As another example, you might have a three-arm trial with placebo, low-dose, and high-dose groups. You want to compare placebo against low dose and you also want to compare it against high dose. You would like to be able to declare a positive study if either comparison is positive. There are several ways to analyze the comparisons, but one way is to allocate an alpha of 0.025 to the comparison between placebo and low dose and the remaining alpha of 0.025 to the comparison between placebo and high dose. This results in two primary endpoints without violating the conventions for Type I error because $0.025 + 0.025 = 0.05$.

It is important to note that, in this case, the p values must be less than 0.025 in order to be able to declare the comparison statistically significant. If, for example, the first comparison between the placebo and low-dose groups yields a p value of 0.03, this would not be statistically significant. If the comparison between the placebo and high-dose groups yields a p value of 0.01, this comparison would be statistically significant.

Much of the statistics for adaptive trial analysis have roots in the techniques for alpha allocation methodologies developed for multiple endpoints, so it is illustrative to examine those techniques.

3.6 Methodologies for Allocating Alpha

3.6.1 Bonferroni Correction

The simplest way to allow multiple comparisons is to split the alpha, by simply dividing 0.05 by the number of endpoints or comparisons, as described above. This type of alpha allocation or correction is called *Bonferroni correction*. Bonferroni correction is often used with *t* tests. So if there are three *t* tests, the *p* value needed for statistical significance is 0.05 divided by 3, or 0.0167. When you perform the statistical test, if the *p* value for one or more of the comparisons is 0.0167 or less, then the study is positive. Otherwise, the study is negative. So, for example, if the *p* values are 0.02, 0.02, and 0.02, the study would be negative for all the comparisons and endpoints.

Bonferroni correction tends to be conservative. If you have more than a handful of *t* tests, you will tend to underestimate significance. The more comparison you do, the worse it will be, because it does not account for double counting—if you already have had a false-positive result, you do not make things worse by having additional false results.

The reason why Bonferroni is conservative is as follows. If you perform pairwise tests such as the *t* test on two arms of a study, they only take into account information from the two arms and ignore that there are other arms. The way a *t* test works is as follows. A *t* test compares the observed variability in each of the two samples (the two arms) against the variability derived from pooling the data from both samples. The idea is that if there is no difference between the two arms, it should not matter whether the variability is calculated from each group or from both groups pooled together. If the variabilities are different, then it suggests that the sample/arms are not in fact similar.

When only one *t* test is performed on the results of a study, that is appropriate. However, for multiple comparisons, it does not take into account all available information. For example, let's say that you are analyzing a study with four arms, A, B, C, and D. The first comparison you do is between A and B. You use the variability data from patients in A and B but not in C and D. You find that there is no difference between A and B. Then you perform a comparison between B and C. With Bonferroni correction, you do not use data from group A. But, in fact, you have information from more than two arms that will give you a better idea of what the total variability or the spread of values should be. You have already determined that A and B groups are equivalent, so you could compare variability in group B and group C against the variability from combined groups A/B/C. There are data from the previous tests but you are not using them in the pairwise tests. You are calculating the numerator and denominator from just two arms when in fact you could use information from all the arms for the denominator. This is why simple

Bonferroni correction is more conservative (less likely to detect a real difference) than other tests.

Also, there is some information carryover. If you compare arm A with arm B and then compare arm B with arm C, you will have some information about arm A vs. arm C by extrapolation. Tests like the *t* test do not take this into consideration.

You can make the tests a little less conservative by modifying the *t* test so that it uses information from all of the arms to estimate the expected spread of the values rather than just from the two arms being compared, but this will only help slightly. This is because the *t* test is designed for comparing groups from studies with only two arms.

Why Bonferroni Is Overly Conservative: By the Numbers

The risk of Type I error when you have three comparisons is as follows. If you just use 0.05 as the cutoff for significance, then with each comparison, you have a 95% chance that you will not draw a false conclusion. So the probability you will not draw a false-positive conclusion is $0.95 \times 0.95 \times 0.95$, which is 0.86. The probability that you will have one or more false positives is 0.14. The Bonferroni method calculates this probability as $0.05 \times 3 = 0.15$. So the values are relatively close.

The risk of Type I error for ten comparisons is as follows. The likelihood that you will not draw a false-positive conclusion is $(0.95)^{10}$, which is 0.60. The Bonferroni method calculates this probability as $0.05 \times 10 = 0.5$. So the difference is much larger.

3.6.2 Holm Correction

The Holm *t* test is less conservative than the Bonferroni correction and is relatively easy to use. You start by ordering the *p* values for each comparison you want to do, from smallest to largest. You sequentially test each comparison, except instead of using 0.05 divided by the number of comparisons as in the Bonferroni correction, you use 0.05 divided by (number of comparisons – number of comparisons you have already performed). So for the first comparison in the example above, you use 0.05/3, but if that is significant, you then use 0.05/2 followed by 0.05/1. You keep on going until you get a result that is not significant. As you can see, this is less conservative than the Bonferroni method because the *p* values are larger.

3.6.3 Other Methods

The other way of performing multiple comparisons is the use of Tukey's test or the Student-Newman-Keuls (SNK) test. Tukey's test, also known as the *Tukey's range test, Tukey's method,* or *Tukey's honestly significant difference test,* is a single-step multiple comparison procedure and statistical test that compares the means of every treatment to the means of every other treatment. In effect, it applies the test simultaneously to the set of all pairwise comparisons.

You start the test by comparing the largest mean value from all of the arms with the smallest mean value from all of the arms. If there is no statistically significant difference between the two means that have the largest difference, comparing any two means that have a smaller difference will yield a negative result unless the sample sizes are different. If there is a difference, you then compare the second largest mean with the smallest mean, and then the next smallest, and so on. Tukey's method is overly conservative when there are unequal sample sizes.

The SNK test is very similar to Tukey's test, except it is less conservative. The SNK test is derived from Tukey's test and is similar except that whereas Tukey's test uses data from all of the groups in the whole study to compute the p value table, the SNK test only uses the groups being compared. In other words, it is more specific in how it calculates the denominator, so that its ability to show a difference is enhanced.

These corrections and tests are very helpful when performing multiple comparisons. In some cases, though, you may not be interested in every pairwise comparison. You might have placebo, old drug, and new drug in the three different arms. You might only be interested in (1) placebo vs. new drug and (2) old drug vs. new drug but not placebo vs. old drug. You do not have to split the alpha across three tests then. Or, in the above example, you only want to know if your drug has an effect or not, and you think both the 5-mg and 10-mg doses will work. Then you can pool the 5-mg and 10-mg groups or use the Dunnett's test, which is a way of comparing many groups and one group.

3.7 Evolution of Adaptive Analytic Methods: Interim Analysis

Eventually, the techniques developed for multiple comparisons led to the development of techniques for interim analysis. Conceptually, traditional interim analysis can be thought of as a type of multiple comparison, except the comparisons are divided across time rather than across endpoints. In other words, rather than performing the test on two or more endpoints, the tests are being performed on the same endpoint except with a different number of patients in the database.

In an interim analysis, an independent data safety monitoring board (DSMB) examines the unblinded data. Based on prespecified criteria, which are specified by the protocol and the statistical analysis plan (SAP), the DSMB makes a recommendation whether to continue or stop the trial. The protocol can specify that the DSMB can stop the trial for safety reasons,

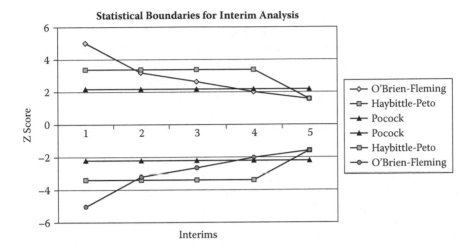

FIGURE 3.1
Stopping boundaries. (Reproduced from R. Chin, *Principles and Practice of Clinical Trial Medicine.* With permission.)

overwhelming efficacy, and/or futility. The prespecified criteria should outline how the statistical analysis will be done and what level of confidence the data must meet in order for the DSMB to act. These criteria must be constructed so that the amount of alpha that is spent by the DSMB plus the alpha spent by the final analysis at the end of the study for efficacy do not add up to more than 0.05.

There are several analytic techniques and procedures for performing interim analysis. The most conventional way is to have a predetermined number of interim analyses and prespecified timing for them. This is called *repeated significance tests*. It essentially means that part of the alpha is spent on (or allocated to) the interim analysis, so that at the end of the study, the combined alpha of the interim analysis plus the final analysis does not exceed 0.05. The three most commonly used techniques are Pocock, Haybittle–Peto, and O'Brien–Fleming, as illustrated in Figure 3.1 (Chin 2008). The differences among the three techniques mostly concern how much of the alpha is spent and when.

Pocock's method, which was one of the first described, uses an equal amount of alpha for each interim analysis. At each interim analysis, if the prespecified significance is met, then the study is stopped. The prespecified significance level is identical for each analysis. So, for example, if there are five analyses, the p value might be 0.01 at each analysis.

The limitation of Pocock's method is that at the beginning of the study, there are fewer patients, and therefore the strength of statistical evidence is lower. With a smaller number of patients, the range of possible values is wider and therefore the probability of spurious results is greater if the significance level is equivalent at each analysis.

With the O'Brien–Fleming method, the statistical penalty is not as great at the beginning of the study. In other words, at the early interim analysis, the results have to be extremely compelling in order to trigger termination of the study. With each subsequent analysis, the boundaries (the p value necessary to trigger termination of the study) become lower and lower.

A limitation of the O'Brien–Fleming approach and similar methods is that the number and timing of the scheduled analysis must be predetermined. In most cases, the analysis must occur at regular and equal intervals. In other words, if the study has 500 patients, the interim analysis may occur every 100 patients or every 125 patients but not at 50, 100, 400, and 500 patients. The statistical algorithms that are used to produce the stopping boundaries do not easily allow, in their unmodified construction, for unequal intervals or changes in the number of interim analyses.

A more flexible methodology is that of Lan–Demets (DeMets and Lan 1994), which allows flexible timing and number of analyses, called the *alpha spending function*. In this approach, the amount of alpha you spend is dependent on the number of patients enrolled (or percentage of study completed, if the study is a time-to-event study) at the time of analysis. The further along the study you are, the more alpha you spend. The timing and the number of interim analyses are much more flexible. The shape of the alpha spending function can be adapted in a flexible manner to the need of the study, as long as the total alpha remains below 0.05.

Of course, the O'Brien–Fleming boundary shape can be implemented as an alpha spending function. It is not uncommon to take the shape of the O'Brien–Fleming boundary and implement it as an alpha spending function. This preserves the ability to impose a high bar for trial termination at the beginning of the study while adding the flexibility to perform the analysis at any time desired. It should be noted that in exchange for the added flexibility, some statistical power is lost when the highly flexible alpha spending function is used. Tsiatis and Mehta (2003) in fact demonstrated that a group sequential technique (discussed later) is theoretically always more powerful than an adaptive study. This paper, however, has been widely misinterpreted, in that although a group sequential technique is always more powerful in theory, in practice you would have to have an interim analysis after every patient in order to exploit that power. Therefore, the additional statistical power afforded by the group sequential technique is largely theoretical.

The most flexible statistical approach to interim analysis is that by Wald, called a *boundaries approach*, which allows for selection between two alternative hypotheses on the basis of the interim looks.

Typically, interim analyses are performed by an independent statistician, who should be someone other than the regular study statistician. The independent statistician should not communicate the interim analysis results to the sponsor or any of the personnel involved in conducting the trial. The results should go only to the independent data monitoring board, unless the interim analysis is being performed for administrative reasons such as initiating another study on the basis of the interim results.

3.8 Adaptive Methods

With the frequentist method, the sample space, or the range of possible outcomes, must be identified in advance so that a p value can be computed. Recall that the frequentist method relies on enumerating all possible outcomes of the study in order to determine how rare the observed results are compared to all possible results. With traditional methods discussed in the last section, this enumeration is possible, and the boundaries defined by the various interim analysis techniques preserve the alpha.

However, the work describe above has been advanced by additional relatively new statistical techniques that are much more powerful and flexible.

Proschan and Hunsberger (1995) described one of the major technical breakthroughs that have enabled adaptive designs. They introduced a technique for using a conditional error function. A *conditional error function* is a function (or a curve) that defines how many additional patients should be enrolled after the interim analysis. The conditional error function is prespecified and described at the beginning of the study. It specifies how much larger the study will need to be under each set of circumstance. At each interim analysis, an *unblinded* analysis is performed to determine the effect size of the treatment. The effect size determines the additional number of patients who will need to be enrolled to attain sufficient power, which is specified by the error function defined at the beginning of the study. Importantly, despite the unblinded examination of the interim data, data from all patients can be used for the final analysis.

The conditional error function is essentially a generalized form of the earlier interim analysis techniques. To put it another way, the previous techniques for generating the stopping boundaries can be considered to be specific instances of the more general conditional error function technique. Rather than calculating the alpha spending for one or more specific points in the study, the conditional error function defines a formula that determines the appropriate amount of alpha that should be spent, depending on when the interim analysis is performed and the result of the analysis.

Another critical statistical milestone in the development of adaptive clinical trials occurred in 1994 when Bauer and Köhne published an influential paper introducing p value combinations. Drawing upon techniques previously used to combine data from multiples studies for meta-analysis, they proposed that there is a way to combine p values from different stages of the same study by weighting the p values appropriately.

For example, you could assign 20% weight to the first 100 patients, perform analysis at that point, and then assign 80% weight to the rest of study, perform the rest of the study, and combine the results. There is a very important distinction between weighting parts of the study versus splitting the alpha. The Bauer method does not so much split the alpha as essentially divide the study into two or more parts. The nominal p values from the various parts are weighted and combined to yield the combined alpha, which is then tested for significance. This conceptual approach of segregating the parts of the study was revolutionary in that alpha could be preserved even if the study was changed on the basis of the interim data.

The advantage of this technique, that the second part of the study can be modified after the first stage, is enormously powerful. This highly adaptive approach goes significantly beyond previous techniques and is sometimes termed *flexible clinical trial design* rather than *adaptive clinical trial design*.

Taken to its logical conclusions, this approach of combining p values is infinitely flexible. In fact, it could allow for completely open design for the second and subsequent stages of the study. In other words, if the study can be divided into two pseudo-independent stages, there is no reason why each stage cannot be further subdivided. And because the second stage is pseudo-independent, the design of the second stage does not have to be pre-specified at the beginning of the study. As long as the first stage is prespecified at the initiation of the study as to the design and weighting, Type I error can be preserved.

There are several implementations of the Bauer method. The first implementation, proposed by Bauer himself and extended by Wassmer, relies on Fisher's combination rule (Fisher 1925). This technique combines the p values based on the fact that $-2 \ln(p)$ for a uniformly distributed p is chi-square distributed. You can therefore obtain a combined test statistic fairly easily using this technique. In other words, combining nominal p values from the various stages of the study can be performed fairly easily because when combined in a specific way the results tend to follow a certain defined pattern.

Other techniques for combining p values exist, including the method by Lechmacher and extended by Cui (1999). The newer approaches allow stopping rules at interim analysis, unlike the original Fisher-based method. The details of the techniques are technical, but they are conceptually similar to the Bauer method. Though they allow for a change in sample size based on unblinded data, these techniques require the number of interim analyses and the way of calculating the combined p value to be declared in advance.

However, the field of adaptive designs has been developing rapidly, and there are several new procedures that add additional flexibility. Shen and Fisher have developed a procedure called *variance spending* that allows not only changes in sample size but also the number of additional interim analysis and relative weightings of the information in the future analyses (Fisher 1998). Essentially, the technique allows continuation of the study and modification at each step based on the previously accumulated data. This technique as originally proposed does not allow for stopping rules until the alpha has been exhausted.

Hartung and Knapp (2003) have developed a more generalized version of the Fisher's combination rule and, using their technique, it is possible to change the relative weighting and number of future analyses.

Both of these techniques are recursive techniques. Whereas the initial techniques divided the study into two or more stages, the newer techniques apply the initial techniques to each stage as if each stage were a study. The recursive techniques therefore allow unlimited application of these techniques to add additional stages as necessary. In other words, if a study can be divided into two or more stages, then the same principle could be applied at the transition from one stage to the next to design additional stages into the remaining stages.

This means that only the first stage needs to be designed at the beginning of the study. Each subsequent stage can be regarded as a blank slate, and as long as the weighting of the next stage is prespecified along with the study design, all stages past the next immediate stage can be left open.

This flexible approach pioneered by Bauer and others has been controversial. Burman and Sonesson (2006) severely criticized it as violating fundamental principles of statistics, including the inference principle, sufficiency principle, invariance principle, and conditionality principle. These criticisms revolve around several issues. First, the order of the stages has an impact on the final result—the exact same clinical data, if the order of patients and stages were reversed, could result in different conclusions. In other words, it makes a difference in the result if the more responsive patients are enrolled in the beginning of the study versus the end of the study.

One example they provided, with modification, is as follows:

> Assume that the interest lies in testing a hypothesis in a study. With 1000 patients at a level of $\alpha = 5\%$, and thus a critical limit $C\alpha = \Phi - 1(1 - \alpha) = 1.645$ for Z. This sample size gives a power of 81% if mean value for the primary endpoint (μ) is 0.08 and standard deviation (σ) = 1.
>
> After 100 patients, it is decided to take an interim look at the data. Disappointingly, the observed average effect is slightly negative, -0.03. The total weight for stage 1 is 0.1, because the sample size was originally planned to be 1000. Assuming that only one more stage will be carried out, the second stage will therefore have the weight $v2 = 1 - v1 = 0.9$.
>
> If the experiment is continued according to plan with 900 patients in the second stage, the power, given the observations from stage 1, is now only 71% under the assumption that the true mean for the endpoint is 0.08, as compared to the original 81%. Several authors have suggested that the sample size modification could be based on a combination of the originally anticipated effect and the observed average. It might be that the experimenter does not find it worthwhile to continue the experiment as planned with 900 patients.

Consider instead the alternative of taking only one single patient in stage 2. For $\mu = 0$, 0.05, and 0.08, for example, the conditional power will then be 3.3%, 3.7%, and 4.0%, respectively. If the experimenter is keen on finding a significant result, this chance may be worth taking. If the observed value of *the next patient* happens to be 2.5, then Thus, the hypothesis test is clearly significant and it is concluded that $\mu > 0$. However, the average of the observations is -0.005.

We have the counterintuitive situation of concluding that the study is positive although the average of the observations is negative. This is due to the different weighting of the observations taken in the study and illustrates the danger of violating the inference principles (Burman 2006).

To summarize, even though the mean change in the mean for the endpoint is -0.005, the conclusion is that the drug works because the 101st patient had a response of 2.5 and his data had nine times more weight than the other 100 patients put together.

This is clearly a counterintuitive result, although to a clinician it is no more counterintuitive than intent-to-treat analysis or Simpson's paradox. There are many nonintuitive concepts and results that are nearly universally accepted in clinical trials today. For example, patients who are randomized to an arm but never receive any doses of the drug or placebo because they drop out of the study immediately. Those patients must be included in the intent-to-treat analysis. Nonetheless, the FDA has been quite wary of accepting these cutting-edge types of adaptive trial designs.

A somewhat less controversial, although still not widely accepted, technique for adaptive designs is the conditional rejection probability technique, developed by Muller and Shafer (2001). This is a hybrid approach. They start from the traditional group sequential design but, using the recursion principle, permit modification of future interim analysis with regard to the sample size, number of future interim analyses, and boundaries for the future interim analyses.

The technique is based on the fact that at each interim analysis, the subsequent period after the interim analysis can be regarded formally as another study, albeit with smaller alpha, and the subsequent stage can be designed relatively freely, just as at the beginning of the study. This approach is somewhat more conservative and avoids some of the issues outlined above with the Bauer technique.

All of the above techniques allow for wide latitude in the design of subsequent stages. Of course, the latitude does not need to be exercised—the decision tree or function can be defined at the beginning of the study. In other words, at the beginning of the study, rules can be specified such that at each interim analysis the decisions made about subsequent stages are driven by the rules prespecified at the beginning of the study. Such designs are called *self-designing studies*.

Another technique that has been developed for interim analysis is the repeated confidence interval method. With multiple interim looks, there is inflation of error in the confidence interval, just as there is with p values. For example, let's say that a study incorporates three interim analyses, and at each interim analysis the 95% confidence interval (CI) is calculated. The likelihood that the actual value is contained within the 95% CI at each interim analysis is 95%. However, the likelihood that the actual value lies within the confidence interval for all three of the interim looks is less than 95%. Specifically, if you perform three interim looks, the likelihood that the actual value is within the 95% CI for all three analyses is $0.95 \times 0.95 \times 0.95 = 0.86$. A method for adjusting the CI to account for this can be used to construct the boundaries for the interim analysis. The method incorporates the number of interim analyses to adjust the boundaries. If the observed value crosses this adjusted boundary, the study can be stopped. Conceptually, this method is in some ways analogous to the stopping boundaries constructed on the basis of adjusted p values discussed above (O'Brien–Fleming, Pocock, etc.).

3.9 Limitations of Adaptive Statistical Techniques

There are several unresolved issues around, and limitations of, adaptive statistical technique, especially the truly flexible designs based on Bauer's technique.

First, although the techniques for group sequential designs and analysis have been well worked out, having been in use since the 1970s, the newer flexible designs are still being invented, debated, and changed. The statistical techniques are still controversial, and the frequentist approach to statistics is poorly suited for the new techniques. It is possible that fundamental underpinnings of frequentist and other statistical approaches may need to be reassessed, a process that will not be quick.

Second, the flexible designs, especially if the endpoint or the patient population is changed, make interpretation of the study results difficult. For example, let's say that the first stage of the study used hospitalization as the endpoint and the second stage used intensive care unit (ICU) hospitalization as the endpoint. If the study is positive (the combined p value is less than 0.05), then the conclusion is that the drug *either reduces hospitalizations or reduces ICU hospitalizations*. The null hypothesis that is rejected is as follows: the drug in the first stage does not reduce hospitalizations AND the drug in the second stage does not reduce ICU hospitalizations. Clearly, the interpretation of such a result can be challenging and confusing.

To be fair, this type of quandary is not unique to flexible designs. Even in a conventional study, inclusion and exclusion criteria or other factors are frequently altered. The conclusion from such studies, to be fair, can also be somewhat unclear. For example, let's say that in the first half of a study for an antianginal drug, patients who had a history of myocardial infarction were excluded, but not in the second. The null hypothesis that is being tested is as follows: the drug does not reduce angina in patients with AND without a prior history of myocardial infarctions. The conclusion, if the study is positive, would be that the drug may work in either both or one of the two study populations but that it is not ineffective in both.

Or to take a slightly more complicated but not an unrealistic example, let's say that the manufacturing process was also altered at the same time as the exclusion criteria was modified. Then the null hypothesis that is being tested is as follows: the first form of the drug does not reduce angina in patients with AND the second form of the drug does not reduce angina without a prior history of myocardial infarctions. The conclusion, if the study is positive, would be that

- The first form of the drug works in patients with no history of myocardial infarction and the second form of the drug works in patients with a history of myocardial infarction.

or

- The first form of the drug works in patients with no history of myocardial infarction and the second form of the drug does not work in patients with a history of myocardial infarction.

or

- The first form of the drug does not work in patients with no history of myocardial infarction and the second form of the drug works in patients with a history of myocardial infarction.

but not

- The first form of the drug does not work in patients with no history of myocardial infarction and the second form of the drug does not work in patients with a history of myocardial infarction.

Interpretation can become complicated even for conventional studies. Of course, subgroup analysis can help disentangle some of these issues.

A third issue is that many of the techniques are better suited for one-sided tests. This means that if the outcome goes in opposite directions at different stages of the study, they may cancel each other out or, more clinically problematic, that a drug that appears to both improve and worsen a disease may result in a positive study. Although appropriate techniques are available to address the first of these problems satisfactorily, the second can be problematic to resolve.

A fourth issue is that with some of these techniques, there must be statistical independence between analyses performed at each stage. The analysis must be carefully planned to avoid potential contamination.

The fifth issue is that because there will be a tendency to select outcomes that appear more likely to work at each decision point, it may be difficult to estimate the magnitude of the effect. For example, let's say that in a study of a drug for asthma, at the first interim analysis the number of hospitalizations seems to be reduced in the active group. The primary endpoint is changed to frequency of hospitalizations and the results are positive. The frequency of hospitalization over the entire study is likely to be overestimated, because, of course, the endpoints selected are going to be the ones that look the most promising at the time of the interim analysis. If the estimate of hospitalizations is based on both stages of the study, then the number from the first stage is probably going to inflate the estimate.

3.10 Bayesian Approach

The Bayesian approach, as mentioned before, can be used in adaptive designs. With Bayesian methods, a distribution of probabilities, called *prior distribution*, is combined with new data to produce a new modified distribution of probabilities, called *posterior distribution*. In many ways, the Bayesian approach is better suited to adaptive designs than the frequentist approach because it can take advantage of real-time data and multiple interim analyses can be performed without the problem of inflation of Type I error.

However, the biggest limitation of the Bayesian approach has been difficulties with the determination of prior probability distribution, which is highly subjective. It may be very difficult to ascertain with any confidence what the likelihood is that a drug is effective. Drug development is a highly risky endeavor, and if it were possible to be relatively certain of success or failure of any drug, the attrition rate for drug candidates would not be 90%.

Frequentist and Bayesian methods are not exactly parallel. Unlike the frequentist approach, which is really a way of drawing conclusions, the Bayesian method is a technique for modifying the data. Frequentist methods allow for drawing conclusions from a set of data. Bayesian methods allow modification of estimates based on data. As an analogy, the frequentist approach will tell you what the price of something is—such as a car. A Bayesian approach will give you a way of paying for the car, such as cash, check, or credit card. It turns out that paying by credit card is much more suited for adaptive clinical trials but, ultimately, the price is better reflected by the price tag on the vehicle.

There have been some attempts to merge frequentist and Bayesian approaches, which to date have been unsuccessful for the most part, satisfying neither the frequentists nor Bayesians.

3.11 Simulations and Modeling

Adaptive clinical trials can become very complicated. This complication can extend to design, execution, and analysis. Fortunately, with modern computers, it is possible to use simulations to plan the studies and to calculate the appropriate adaptations during the study. In many cases, this is essential, because the number of permutations that an adaptive trial can grow into can be very large or infinite. Though the strength of adaptive designs is that the study can change quite a bit during the execution, the challenge is that because it can vary so much, the potential range of changes must be estimated in advance so that appropriate budget, drug supply, and other practical arrangements can be made. Otherwise, the study may run out of drug, time, or personnel. In addition, though the exact course of the study cannot be known, it is important to have assurances that the size and the cost of the study will not be impractical.

Simulation is the process of running multiple iterations of a mathematical model meant to imitate a real-life process, such as a study. Essentially, clinical simulations are virtual experiments to test the effects of changing different parameters and of testing random variation on results of a study.

The alternative to a simulation would be to comprehensively calculate every possible variation of the study, but in many cases that is too complicated and numerous even for modern computers. In rare instances, however, that is possible, and these are called *deterministic models*. Deterministic models provide the same answer every time you run the model. In other words, the model variables and parameters are fixed, that is, constant or the same each time. A deterministic model can provide exact predictions on the likelihood of each outcome rather than an approximate prediction.

Simulations are stochastic (probabilistic) models and they incorporate uncertainty into the model. The key parameters are uncertain and may change every time you run the model. The parameters can be programmed to vary completely randomly, with a normal variation, in an exponential fashion, in a Poisson distribution, or in some other fashion. Typically, after several thousand or million iterations, a pattern emerges that should approximate what will happen with the real study.

One common example of a stochastic model is the Monte Carlo simulation. In a Monte Carlo simulation, key variables are drawn from a probabilistic distribution and results also come in the form of a distribution. For example, it may incorporate a certain probability that a drug will improve outcome by 10, 20, and 30%. And based on that and other probability distributions, the model can predict how likely it is that the study will stop after the first interim, second interim, or third interim analysis.

Another alternative to simulation is the expected value model. With this technique, the likelihood of each possible chain of events is calculated by assigning a value to each possible outcome. The outcome values are combined to yield the expected value. In other words, if there is a sequence of five events, each with two outcomes, then any particular set of five events can be calculated by multiplying the probability of each outcome for each event. Though this technique gives a reasonable guess as to the most likely outcome, it does not give good information about the distribution of other possible outcomes around the expected value.

When you do not know the probability distribution, a method called bootstrapping can be used. With this technique, you generate the probability distribution from the model itself. It is a bit counterintuitive, but you take the model and from it take a number of iterations of the model. Essentially, the model generates a distribution based on some initial runs of the simulation. Based on these data, a distribution model is calculated and then fed back into the simulation.

For adaptive studies, various ways of changing the parameters of the study can be fed into the simulation. The parameters can specify multiple types of decision trees and boundaries. For example, the simulation can be run with a stopping boundary of 0.01 at the first interim analysis and 0.02 at the second interim, or it can be run with a boundary of 0.001 at the first interim and 0.005 at the second interim. The model can predict the likelihood that the study would be stopped at each interim analysis given the stopping boundaries. This can yield a reasonable estimate of how the results might vary, as well point the way toward the optimal number of interim analyses, timing of the analyses, etc. The sponsor can predict what the likelihood is that additional resources may be needed, what the likelihood is that more clinical supplies will be required, and so forth.

There are multiple other uses for the simulations. Some examples, as enumerated by the FDA for modeling, include models for study endpoints or outcomes, models for the withdrawal or dropout of subjects, and models of the procedure for selecting among multiple study endpoints (FDA 2010). There can also be models for event rate background, subgroup differences, or heterogeneity in response. Extensive modeling is sometimes required to plan and design the study appropriately.

3.12 The FDA's Stance on Adaptive Techniques

The FDA divides the statistical techniques discussed above into two categories: generally well-understood adaptive designs and adaptive designs whose properties are less well understood. They are comfortable with the first and not as comfortable with the second. Their perspective is excerpted below (FDA 2010) FDA's draft guidance on adaptive trials.

V. GENERALLY WELL-UNDERSTOOD ADAPTIVE DESIGNS WITH VALID APPROACHES TO IMPLEMENTATION

There are well-established clinical study designs that have planned modifications based on an interim study result analysis (perhaps multiple times within a single study) that either need no statistical correction related to the interim analysis or properly account for the analysis-related multiplicity of choices. Considerable experience in modern drug development provides confidence that these design features and procedures will enhance efficiency while limiting the risk of introducing bias or impairing interpretability.

Many of the best understood adaptive design methods do not involve examining unblinded study outcome data and examine only aggregate study outcome data, baseline data, or data not related to the effectiveness outcome (see sections V.A, B, and C). Other adaptive methods use the well-understood group sequential design (see section and the ICH E9 guidance). In group sequential designs, unblinded interim analyses of accruing study data are used in a planned and confidential manner (i.e., by a data monitoring committee [DMC]) that controls Type I error and maintains study integrity.

This section will describe some of the approaches that are well understood, emphasizing the principles that explain why they are well understood. The descriptions and discussion in the following subsections are intended to aid in determining whether other existing or future developed methods share the same principles.

A. Adaptation of Study Eligibility Criteria Based on Analyses of Pretreatment

Clinical studies are generally planned with expectations about the patient population characteristics and the rate at which eligible patients will be identified and enrolled. For example, the study designers may have tried to enroll patients with a broad distribution in certain identified characteristics to maximize a study's utility. Examination of baseline characteristics of the accumulating study population might show that the expected population is not being enrolled and that by modifying eligibility criteria, subsequent subject enrollment may be shifted toward a population with greater numbers of patients with the desired characteristics. Similarly, if the study enrollment rate is substantially slower than expected, the screening log can be examined for noncritical entry criteria that might be modified to allow greater numbers of screened patients to qualify.

Such examination of baseline information and modification of study eligibility criteria can contribute to timely completion of informative studies. Knowing the baseline characteristics of the overall study population at any time during the study does not generate concerns of introducing statistical bias as long as the treatment assignment remains blinded.

A possible risk of such an approach is the potential to impair the interpretation of the study result when the study population changes midway and an important relationship of treatment effect to the changed patient characteristic exists (i.e., a treatment–patient factor interaction). Exploratory analyses of the data obtained before and after the eligibility change can help to identify such problems.

Because post-baseline patient data are not involved in the analyses, the study sponsor or investigator steering committee can review the baseline data summaries and make design changes to the eligibility criteria without risk to the integrity of the study.

B. Adaptations to Maintain Study Power Based on Blinded Interim Analyses of Aggregate Data

One of the important challenges in planning adequate and well-controlled (A&WC) studies is deciding on the sample size at the study design stage. In general, the estimated power of a study to detect a treatment effect is dependent upon the study sample size, the targeted (e.g., the sponsor's assumed actual or minimum acceptable) treatment effect size, the assumed population variance of the patient measure being studied, or the expected control group event rate for event-driven studies. If any of the assumptions used to calculate the sample size are incorrect, the study may be underpowered and fail to show an effect. There are several approaches to maintaining study power.

In studies using a discrete outcome (event) endpoint, a blinded examination of the study overall event rate can be compared to the assumptions used in planning the study. Examining the data in this blinded analysis does not introduce statistical bias, and no statistical adjustments are required. If this comparison suggests that the actual event rate is well below the initial assumption, the study will be underpowered. The study sample size can be increased to maintain the desired study power or, alternatively, study duration might be increased to obtain additional endpoint events. Study resizing based on a revised estimate of event rate should be used cautiously early in the study, because variability of the estimated event rate can be substantial. Consequently, this adaptive approach may be best applied later in the study when population estimates of the event rate are more stable.

For studies using a time-to-event analysis, another approach is not to plan a specific study sample size in the protocol but rather to continue patient enrollment until a prospectively specified number of events has occurred (an event-driven study). The interim data analyses are of the overall number of study endpoint events, rather than the overall rate of events.

Similarly, when a continuous outcome measure is the study endpoint, a blinded examination of the variance of the study endpoint can be made and compared to the assumption used in planning the study. If this comparison suggests the initial assumption was substantially too low and the study is consequently underpowered, an increase in the study sample size can maintain the desired study power. As with event endpoints, study resizing based on a revised estimate of variance should be used cautiously early in the study, because variability of the estimated variance can be substantial.

In some studies with continuous outcome measures the duration of patient participation and time of last evaluation may be the preferred design feature to modify. A study of a chronic, progressive disease with a treatment intended to stabilize the clinical status is dependent upon the control group demonstrating a worsening of the condition, but there may have been only limited prior data upon which the design-assumed rate of progression was based. An interim analysis of the aggregate rate of progression can be useful to assess whether the duration of the study should be adjusted to allow for sufficient time for the group responses to be distinguished, given the assumed treatment effect size. A combination of sample size and duration modification can also be applied in this case to maintain the desired study power.

Alternatively, if it is thought that patients can be stratified at baseline (e.g., by a genetic or disease phenotype characteristic) into subsets expected to differ in an important aspect related to the endpoint (e.g., event rate, variance, rate of disease progression), the blinded interim analysis of the event rate (or, e.g., variance) can be done by subset and study eligibility criteria modified to focus the remainder of the study on the subset(s) with the advantageous tendency (e.g., greater event rate, lower variance). A sample size readjustment could be considered at the same time.

Usually, the blinded interim analyses considered here are used to make decisions to increase the sample size but not to decrease the study size. Decreasing sample size is not advisable because of the chance of making a poor choice caused by the high variability of the effect size and event rate or variance estimates early in the study.

The ability of these procedures to increase the potential for a successful study while maintaining Type I error control has been recognized and discussed in the ICH E9 guidance (www.ICH.org). Sample size adjustment using blinded methods to maintain desired study power should generally be considered for most studies.

Because these methods avoid introducing bias by using only blinded interim analyses, all study summaries should not contain any information potentially revealing the between-group differences. For example, even a data display showing the distribution of aggregate interim results might reveal the presence, and suggest a size, of a treatment effect (e.g., a histogram showing a bimodal distribution of the endpoint data) and might influence the personnel making these adaptations.

C. Adaptations Based on Interim Results of an Outcome Unrelated to Efficacy

There are some circumstances where study modifications are based on an interim analysis of outcomes that are independent of, and uninformative about, the treatment-related efficacy effect. Concerns about statistical and operational bias usually are not raised by such interim analyses and modifications if there has been no unblinded analysis of any effectiveness-related data. Control of Type I error rate is thus maintained without a statistical adjustment for such adaptations. At the time that a study is being designed it is not uncommon to be uncertain about how patients may respond to the treatment in ways not measured by the efficacy outcome. For example, there may be a known or potential adverse reaction with an incidence too low to have been accurately estimated from prior experience but of a severity so substantial that it could outweigh the possible benefits from the treatment.

Randomized, parallel dose–response studies are generally most informative when a broad range of doses is studied. When this is done, however, some doses might cause an unacceptable rate of a serious adverse effect or a less serious adverse effect sufficient to make the treatment unattractive (e.g., causing a high treatment discontinuation rate). It is therefore important to look for these events at an interim stage of the study and discontinue a dose group with unacceptable observed toxicity. If the adverse effect is completely independent of the treatment's benefit, then an unblinded analysis of the rate of the adverse effect provides no knowledge of the efficacy results and the Type I error rate remains controlled without an adjustment. Similarly, if an unexpected serious toxicity is observed in safety monitoring, dropping the dose groups with excessive toxicity is usually appropriate.

It is common to have study designs that initiate testing with several dose or regimen groups, with the intent of dropping dose groups that are poorly tolerated and enrolling subsequent patients into the remaining groups. To ensure full awareness of the process and avoid missteps that could compromise the study integrity, the design and analysis plan should specify the number of groups to be terminated, how they will be selected, and the appropriate analysis procedures for testing the final data (e.g., adjustment for multiplicity when more than one dose is planned to be carried to completion). A design of this type may be particularly useful in long-duration studies where the adverse event of concern occurs at a low rate (and therefore cannot be precisely assessed in small exploratory studies) and occurs relatively early after initiating treatment. For example, studies of platelet-inhibiting drugs have sought to demonstrate long-term efficacy using the highest dose not causing excessive rates of early bleeding.

It is important to emphasize that this approach may be undesirable if there might be greater effectiveness associated with the more toxic dose that could outweigh the increased toxicity in a risk–benefit comparison. The nature and implications of the possibly greater toxicity should be carefully considered and this approach used only when there is confidence that the greater toxicity will outweigh greater effectiveness.

If there are no efficacy-related interim analyses performed, the interpretability of the final study result is not impaired by concerns of statistical bias or operational bias in study conduct. Study planning should assure that the personnel who make the modification decision (e.g., a steering committee) have not previously seen any unblinded efficacy analyses. As emphasized, the outcome examined must not be the efficacy outcome or an outcome related to efficacy in any way that allows inferences to be formed regarding the efficacy outcome. Thus, secondary or tertiary efficacy endpoints, or biomarkers thought to have some relationship to efficacy, should not be used in this approach. A design modification based on an efficacy-related endpoint or biomarker will call for an appropriate statistical adjustment (see section VI.C [below]). Situations in which a drug-induced serious or fatal outcome is an event to be avoided (and thus monitored for treatment-related increase) and is also an important component of a composite efficacy outcome cannot be considered in this paradigm. Other approaches (e.g., group sequential designs) should be used in these situations to protect the integrity of the study. The concern is that because the interim results are related to efficacy, the DMC might be biased in making any subsequent decisions about study modification.

D. Adaptations Using Group Sequential Methods and Unblinded Analyses for Early Study Termination because of either Lack of Benefit or Demonstrated Efficacy

Group sequential statistical design and analysis methods have been developed that allow valid analyses of interim data and provide well-recognized alpha spending approaches to address the control of the Type I error rate (e.g., O'Brien–Fleming, Lan-DeMets, Peto methods) to enable termination of a study early when either no beneficial treatment effect is seen or a statistically robust demonstration of efficacy is observed. Aspects of group sequential monitoring are discussed in the ICH E9 guidance.

In circumstances where the drug has little or no benefit, the data accumulated before planned completion of the study might provide sufficient evidence to conclude that the study is unlikely to succeed on its primary objective, even if it were carried to completion. Discontinuing the study for these reasons at this interim point, often called *futility*, might save resources and avoid exposure of more patients to a treatment of no value.

Studies with multiple groups (e.g., multiple dose levels) can be designed to carry only one or two groups to completion out of the several initiated, based on this type of futility analysis done by group. One or more unblinded interim analyses of the apparent treatment effect in each group are examined, and groups that meet the prospective futility criterion are terminated. However, because of the multiplicity arising from the several sequential interim analyses over time with multiple between-group analyses done to select groups to discontinue (see section VI.A [below]), statistical adjustments and the usual group sequential alpha spending adjustments need to be made in this case to control Type I error rates.

For the group sequential methods to be valid, it is important to adhere to the prospective analytic plan, terminating the group if a futility criterion is met and not terminating the study for efficacy unless the prospective efficacy criterion is achieved. Failure to follow the prospective plan in either manner risks confounding interpretation of the study results.

If the drug is more effective than expected, the accumulating data can offer strong statistical evidence of the therapy's success well in advance of the planned completion of the study. If the study outcome is one of great clinical importance, such as survival or avoidance of irreversible disability, ethical considerations may warrant early termination of the study and earlier advancement of the product toward widespread availability in medical practice. It is important to bear in mind that early termination for efficacy should generally be reserved for circumstances in which there is the combination of compelling ethical concern and robust statistical evidence. A study terminated early will have a smaller size than the initially planned study size. It will therefore provide less safety data than planned. A potential also exists for more difficulty with the efficacy analysis and interpretation related to issues that become apparent only during the later detailed analysis (e.g., related to loss to follow-up or debatable endpoint assessments) and decreased power to assess patient subsets of interest.

Group sequential designs offer a method for early termination of a study as an adaptive design element, allowing the study sample size to be reduced to the size accumulated at the time of an interim data analysis. Most of the commonly used methods employ conservative (small p value) criteria for terminating on the basis of demonstrated efficacy.

Implementation of group sequential design methods involves unblinded analyses of the treatment effect, thereby raising significant concerns for potentially introducing bias into the conduct of the study or into subsequent decisions regarding the conduct of the study. Protocols using group sequential designs have addressed this concern by using a committee independent of the study's conduct and sponsor to examine these analyses in a secure and confidential manner. An independent, non-sponsor-controlled DMC (see the DMC guidance [www.FDA.Gov]) is an inherent part of the group sequential method's protection of study integrity. These well-established DMC procedures more recently have led to using DMCs to implement other adaptive procedures as well. Less well settled, however, is which parties prepare the analyses for the DMC to consider and the independence of the statistician preparing these analyses. The DMC guidance does not reach firm conclusions on this, but it is critical that the analyses be carried out either externally to the study sponsor or by a group within the sponsor that is unequivocally separated from all other parties to the study.

An unblinded interim analysis exposes the DMC (or other involved committee) to confidential information. Any subsequent decisions or recommendations by the DMC related to any aspect of study design, conduct, or analysis can be influenced by the knowledge of interim results, even if the decision is intended to be unrelated to the prior interim analysis. For example, if new information should become available from a source outside the study, but relevant to the ongoing study, the DMC will no longer be the appropriate group to consider and recommend study design changes in response to the new information. This task will usually fall to a blinded steering committee. This issue is emphasized in the DMC guidance.

E.   Adaptations in the Data Analysis Plan Not Dependent on Within Study, Between-Group Outcome Differences

The SAP for the clinical trial often makes assumptions regarding the distribution of the outcome data. Analytic methods may also be sensitive to the amount of, or approach to, various types of observed data (e.g., distribution of values, missing data). When study data do not conform to the assumptions of the planned analytic methods or are overly sensitive to other data behavior, the validity of conclusions drawn from the study analysis can be affected.

Generally, the prospective SAP should be written carefully and completely and implemented without further changes once the study has started. However, if blinding has been unequivocally maintained, limited changes to the SAP late in the study can be considered. The ICH E9 guidance suggests that after a blinded inspection of the data, the SAP can be updated regarding the appropriate data transformations, adding covariates identified from other research sources or reconsideration of parametric versus nonparametric analysis methods. In some cases, with unequivocal assurance that unblinding has not occurred, this approach can also be applied to changes in the primary endpoint, composition of the defined endpoint event, or endpoint analytic sequence ordering.

In certain situations, the optimal statistical analysis plan may be difficult to specify fully before completing the study and examining the relevant characteristics of the final outcome data. If these characteristics are examined for the entire study population in a blinded manner, analytic plan modifications based on these characteristics do not introduce bias. The prospective analysis plan should clearly specify the characteristics and the procedure for selecting the analysis methodology based on these data characteristics.

Examples of where this may be useful include situations in which the observed data violate prospective assumptions regarding the distribution of the data or where data transformations or use of a covariate is called for in the analysis to achieve adequate conformity with the method's assumptions.

Adaptation of the primary endpoint according to prospectively specified rules may also be useful in some circumstances. For example, when an outcome assessment that is preferred as the primary endpoint proves difficult to obtain, a substantial amount of missing data may occur for this assessment. An analytic plan might direct that if the amount of missing data in the preferred outcome assessment exceeds some prospectively stated criterion, a specified alternative outcome would be used as the primary efficacy endpoint. Similarly, when a composite event endpoint is used but there is uncertainty regarding the event rates to expect for the possible components, an analytic plan accommodating inclusion of one or two specific additional types of events might be appropriate if an insufficient number of events within the initial composite were observed in the overall study. In a similar manner, selection or sequential order of secondary endpoints might also be adapted.

VI. ADAPTIVE STUDY DESIGNS WHOSE PROPERTIES ARE LESS WELL UNDERSTOOD

This section provides an overview of adaptive study designs with which there is relatively little regulatory experience and whose properties are not fully understood at this time. These clinical trial design and statistical analysis methods are primarily intended for circumstances where the primary study objective(s) cannot be achieved by other study designs, such as those described in section V. The study design and analysis methods discussed in this section are limited to parallel group randomized study designs, and they can have several adaptive stages. The chief concerns with these designs are control of the study-wide Type I error rate, minimization of the impact of any adaptation-associated statistical (see section VII.B) or operational bias on the estimates of treatment effects, and the interpretability of trial results. This section does not discuss sequential group dose escalation study designs or dose deescalation study designs, which are noncomparative designs that can be conducted in early drug development.

The less well-understood adaptive design methods are all based on unblinded interim analyses that estimate the treatment effect(s). The focus of the discussions in this section is primarily on specific categories of adaptation methods, whereas the more general implementation issues that the methods raise are discussed in section VII.

A. Adaptations for Dose Selection Studies

A critical component of drug development is to estimate the shape and location of the dose–response relationship for effectiveness and adverse effects, which can have different dose relationships. Understanding these relationships facilitates selecting doses for more definitive effectiveness and safety evaluation in the A&WC studies of late clinical development (see the FDA's ICH E4 guidance *on Dose–Response Information to Support Drug Registration* [at www.FDA.Gov]), and in some cases can provide labeling guidance on starting and maximum doses for patient management.

Too often, however, the A&WC studies evaluate only a single dose or two doses spanning a narrow dose range based on a tenuously understood dose–response relationship developed from very limited data. Unsuccessful development can result from focusing on a single dose in the A&WC studies if the single selected dose does not demonstrate effectiveness or if very important but less common adverse effects are identified in the larger A&WC studies, whereas a different dose could have provided an improved benefit to risk comparison. It is also possible that the selected dose is needlessly large and the excessive dose causes a serious but uncommon adverse effect that will be discovered only in the postmarketing period. Consequently, there is considerable interest in whether adaptive design techniques based on unblinded interim analysis of efficacy data can enable improved understanding of the dose–response relationship.

The term *dose* refers not only to a specific chosen dose level but also includes the schedule (i.e., administration frequency) and in some cases the duration of use. The different doses evaluated in a dose–response study can be distinguished by any of these aspects of a regimen. Typically, a dose exploration study randomizes patients among placebo and several dose groups. The resulting data can be analyzed to identify the one or several groups with best response (i.e., the existence of a dose–response relationship for effectiveness or safety) or for the therapeutic window (by balancing safety, including tolerability, and efficacy).

An adaptive exploratory dose–response study is intended to begin with multiple doses (sometimes many) across a range. The number of dose groups is adaptively decreased during the course of the study, using the accruing efficacy or safety data in a prospectively specified plan for design modification at one or more unblinded interim analyses. The response evaluated at the interim analyses is often the clinical efficacy endpoint but could also be a biomarker. Many adaptive study designs only eliminate unsuitable or uninformative doses, but addition of new, potentially more preferable, doses is also possible. Some adaptive designs can also adjust the sample size of the overall study or of the individual dose groups to obtain response estimates of a particular desired precision. In some situations, an exposure–response relationship for effectiveness or safety may be used in place of dose–response. These prospectively planned study designs offer flexibility that can allow many potential modifications.

A particularly interesting exploratory approach is to use an adaptive design exploratory dose–response study with a moderate number of doses (five to seven) with the objective of identifying the shape (from among several different potential modeled-shape relationships) and location of the dose–response relationship, as well as optimizing selection of two or three doses (which might be the same as, or between, doses that were tested in the exploratory study) for evaluation in subsequent A&WC studies. Irrespective of whether this particular approach is used, fully evaluating more than one dose in the larger A&WC studies is almost always advisable whenever feasible.

Highly flexible modifications should generally be limited to an exploratory study, but some of these approaches, when used with rigorous protection of the Type I error rate, might have a role in A&WC studies. For example, a common design for an A&WC study is to evaluate two doses thought likely to offer a favorable benefit–risk comparison. If there was significant residual uncertainty in selecting the two doses, the study design might also include a third dose to begin the study (higher or lower than the two doses thought likely). An interim analysis of the treatment effect in each dose group would enable terminating the dose that appeared least likely to be useful, allowing the study to continue thorough evaluation of two doses with improved chances for success. Using this approach in an A&WC study will call for careful statistical adjustment to control the Type I error rate and should be limited to modest pruning of the number of dose groups.

In some development programs a biomarker (or an endpoint other than a clinical effectiveness endpoint) might be used for the interim analysis to determine the adaptive modification. If there is limited or uncertain predictiveness of the biomarker for the clinical outcome, however, there may be uncertainty regarding how well such a design will optimize the drug's clinical effects. Sponsors should consider the level of uncertainty in that relationship and the potential consequences when planning to employ this approach. In addition, because of the correlation between the biomarker and the ultimate clinical endpoint, introduction of bias is a concern and statistical adjustments are needed to control the Type I error rate.

B. Adaptive Randomization Based on Relative Treatment Group Responses

Adaptive randomization is a form of treatment allocation in which the probability of patient assignment to any particular treatment group of the study is adjusted based on repeated comparative analyses of the accumulated outcome responses of patients previously enrolled (often called *outcome dependent randomization;* for example, the "play the winner" approach). The randomization schedule across the study groups can change frequently or continuously over the duration of the study. This design is facilitated when the subjects' outcomes are observed soon after initial exposure relative to the rate at which study enrollment occurs. Previously, this randomization method had been used in placebo controlled studies chiefly to place more patients into the group with better outcomes.

More recently the approach has been revised to suit the objective of dose–response evaluation. The method allocates fewer subjects to doses that appear to have a low probability of a treatment-related efficacy response, to have a high probability of an adverse event, or to be unlikely to contribute additional information on the shape of the dose–response profile. Outcome-dependent adaptive randomization is particularly valuable for exploratory studies because it can make practical an increase in the number of tested treatment options (increased breadth to the range of doses tested and/or decreased step size between doses) explored for the drug's activity and facilitate estimation of the dose–response relationship, and hypothesis testing is not the study objective. Adaptive randomization should be used cautiously in A&WC studies, because the analysis is not as easily interpretable as when fixed randomization probabilities are used. Particular attention should be paid to avoiding bias and controlling the Type I error rate.

The expectation in clinical studies of balance among the treatment groups with regard to important baseline characteristics relies upon the use of randomization and provides a valid basis for statistical comparisons. When patient outcome is a function of covariates and treatment group assignment, changing randomization probabilities over the course of the study raises a concern regarding the balance of patient characteristics among the treatment groups. If patients enrolled into the study change in the relevant baseline characteristics (either measured or unmeasured) over the time course of the study, the changing allocation probabilities could lead to poor balance in patient characteristics between the groups at the end of the study. If the characteristics in poor balance have an influence on outcome, inaccuracy is introduced into the estimated treatment effect between groups. A dose–response profile obtained from an exploratory study with this approach could lead to poor dose selection for subsequent studies; this issue should be considered for such studies. Such poor balance in important characteristics could be a very significant problem for an A&WC study. To address the concern regarding patient characteristics, we recommend that sponsors maintain randomization to the placebo group to ensure that sufficient patients are enrolled into the placebo group along the entire duration of the study. Examining an exploratory analysis of response over time within the placebo group and examining exploratory comparisons of response in the placebo group to drug-treated groups by dividing the study into periods of enrollment may help evaluate this concern for a completed study. Maintaining the placebo group will also best maintain the power of the study to show a treatment effect. It is also prudent to consider the treatment effect estimate obtained from an adaptive randomization exploratory study cautiously, and this estimate should probably be used more conservatively in setting the sample size of a subsequent A&WC study to offset the potential overestimate of effect size.

C. Adaptation of Sample Size Based on Interim Effect Size Estimates

In a fixed sample size A&WC study design, planning for the sample size involves consideration of the following: a postulated treatment effect size, an assumption about the placebo event rate in event outcome studies or the variability of the primary outcome endpoint in other studies, the desired Type I error rate, and the desired power to detect the posited treatment effect size. Other factors (e.g., stratification and dropout rates) can also be considered. Usually, the sample size (or total event count) is prospectively determined and fixed in advance using this information; however, study designs with group sequential methodology (see section V.D) might stop the study early with a smaller than planned sample size (or event count) for either lack of effect or overwhelming evidence of an effect larger than expected. Section V.B describes a number of adaptations of sample size or event count (or study duration in certain circumstances) based on blinded analyses. In contrast, one adaptive design approach is to allow an increase in the initially planned study sample size based on knowledge of the unblinded treatment effect sizes at an interim stage of the study if the interim-observed treatment effect size is smaller than had been anticipated but still clinically relevant. In general, using this approach late in the study is not advisable because a large percentage increase in sample size at that point is inefficient. In some designs, other study features that affect the estimated power of the study might be changed at the same time, such as modifying the components of a composite primary endpoint (see section VI.E). In other cases, an adaptation that focuses on another aspect of study design (e.g., dose, population, study endpoint) could alter the study power, warranting reestimation of study sample size to maintain study power. There are several methods for modifying the sample size of the trial, and these methods frequently are based on conditional power or predictive power. Adaptive designs employing these methods should be used only for increases in the sample size, not for decreases. The potential to decrease the sample size is best achieved through group sequential designs with well-understood alpha spending rules structured to accommodate the opportunity to decrease the study size by early termination at the time of the interim analysis.

A change in study sample size related to an unblinded data analysis (as opposed to one based on blinded analyses discussed in section V.B) can cause an increase in the Type I error rate. To protect against such an increase, a statistical adjustment is necessary for the final study analysis.

Some methods for this adjustment decrease the alpha level at which statistical significance is determined, whereas other methods will perform the hypothesis test at the usual alpha level but weight the data from the successive portions of the study unequally. Another method combines aspects of both alpha adjustment and weighting adjustment and generally results in reasonable sample size increases. The weights for each study portion should be selected prospectively and not determined after the unblinded interim analysis. The selected balance of weights should be carefully considered because they can affect the statistical efficiency of the design. Differential weighting, however, can lead to some difficulties in interpreting the final analysis.

When the weighting is not proportional to the patient numbers in each stage, individual patient data from the different stages do not have equal contribution to the overall treatment effect estimate. This could lead to an estimate of the treatment effect that is different from the estimate when all patients are given equal weight, with resulting confusion regarding the amount of benefit demonstrated.

Estimates of treatment effect observed early in the study, when there are relatively fewer patient data, are generally variable and can be misleadingly large or small. Thus, those responsible for monitoring the study should act conservatively when deciding upon study changes using the early estimates. This is similar in spirit to the approach used in group sequential design alpha spending functions, where more conservative alpha spending is used early in the study.

D. Adaptation of Patient Population Based on Treatment Effect Estimates

As previously noted (for blinded analysis methods discussed in section V.B), modification of the patient population enrolled (i.e., enrichment modification designs) into a study can sometimes improve the power of a study to detect a treatment effect. The blinded analysis methods are useful when the purpose of the modification is to increase the ability to show a treatment effect when the treatment effect is not expected to substantially differ among the various population subsets. These methods do not raise concern about increasing the Type I error rate.

In some circumstances, however, genetic, physiologic, or other baseline characteristics are thought to potentially distinguish patient subsets that have differing responsiveness to the drug treatment. Identifying these characteristics is typically done as part of exploratory studies and is important to selecting the patient population for study in the A&WC studies. Adaptive design studies using unblinded interim analyses (of either clinical or biomarker data) for each subset of interest have been proposed as another method for identifying population subsets with relatively greater treatment responsiveness. Adaptive methods might, for example, be used within a traditional dose–response exploratory study so that the study results guide optimal design for dose and population selections for the subsequent A&WC study.

In some cases where the data from exploratory studies are suggestive of population subset response differences but inadequate to confidently select a fixed patient population for the A&WC study, these methods might be cautiously applied in an A&WC study to modify eligibility criteria after the interim analysis. These designs are less well understood, pose challenges in avoiding introduction of bias, and generally call for statistical adjustment to avoid increasing the Type I error rate.

Adaptive methods that have been proposed include (1) changing only the eligibility criteria, with no change in the study overall sample size and with the final analysis including the entire study population; or (2) modifying the plan for the final analysis to include only patients with the preferred characteristic. Other methods can increase the sample size for the population subset with the desired characteristic. The prospective study plan should ensure control of the Type I error rate for all hypotheses tested. Each method will involve different approaches to statistical adjustment. There may be no statistical adjustment necessary if there are no changes in the hypotheses tested. Caution should be exercised in planning studies where an interim analysis and eligibility modification are performed multiple times, because when multiple revisions to the study population are made it may be challenging to obtain adequate estimates of the treatment effect in the populations of interest or to interpret to what patient population the results apply.

E. Adaptation for Endpoint Selection Based on Interim Estimate of Treatment Effect

Planning a clinical trial involves careful selection of the primary and secondary effectiveness endpoints. At the planning stage, the optimal endpoints for assessing the disorder or the disease aspects that best exhibit the particular drug's effects may not be well understood. Choosing endpoints in this circumstance may be difficult at the time of study design.

Changing the ordering of endpoints (including switching primary and secondary endpoints) based on an unblinded interim analysis of treatment effect might have value in such cases.

Endpoint adaptation should have appropriate statistical procedures to control the Type I error rate for the multiplicity of possible endpoint selections. If the size of the interim data set is insufficient to provide a stable assessment of the effect sensitivity differences between endpoints, however, this approach risks selecting a poor endpoint.

Primary endpoint revision usually takes one of two forms, replacement of the designated primary endpoint with an entirely new endpoint or modification of the primary endpoint by adding or removing data elements to the endpoint (e.g., the discrete event types included in a composite event endpoint). In addition to prospectively stating all possible endpoint modifications, study designers should ensure that all possible choices are appropriate for the objective of the study (e.g., all possible primary endpoints in an A&WC study are clinical efficacy endpoints). This adaptive design approach is an alternative to a fixed design with two (or more) primary endpoints and appropriate multiplicity adjustment. Study planners should ensure that the adaptive design provides advantages over the fixed design before adopting it.

A general concern with endpoint modification involves the quality of the data on each endpoint. For example, knowledge of which endpoint has been designated the primary endpoint and/or the chief secondary endpoint could influence the study conduct at some sites in the evaluations for endpoints (or endpoint event components) designated less important (i.e., as only backup endpoints) and lead to lower quality data than for those initially designated most important. An interim analysis that includes these lower quality endpoint data can result in misleading effect size comparisons between endpoints and a counterproductive change in the endpoint. Sponsors conducting an endpoint-adaptive study should be particularly alert to ensuring that the data on each endpoint are collected in a uniform manner with good quality, both before and after the interim analysis and design modification.

F. Adaptation of Multiple-Study Design Features in a Single Study

In theory, adaptive design methods allow more than one design feature to be modified during a study. The study design should prospectively account for the multiple adaptations and maintain control of the study-wide Type I error rate. An adaptive design study could include interim analyses for any of a number of adaptations, such as modification of treatment dose, efficacy endpoint, patient subset, study duration, or study sample size. These revisions could be made at one time or divided across several times during a study.

When multiple adaptations are planned within a single study, the study will become increasingly complex and difficult to plan, with increased difficulty in interpreting the study result. In addition, if there are interactions between the changes in study features, multiple adaptations can be counterproductive and lead to failure of the study to meet its goals.

Because of these concerns, an A&WC study should limit the number of adaptations. Exploratory studies may be better suited to circumstances when multiple adaptations are warranted.

G.   Adaptations in Noninferiority Studies

Noninferiority studies rely on many of the same types of assumptions in determining the study design features that are used to design superiority comparison studies. Accuracy of these assumptions similarly affects whether the study is adequately powered to achieve the study objective. When there is uncertainty in these assumptions, noninferiority studies also have the potential to be strengthened by interim analyses that examine the accuracy of some of these assumptions and readjust the study size, if appropriate. A blinded interim analysis (e.g., of overall event rate, variance, demographic features of the study population) can often be entirely sufficient to enable reconsideration of study sample size (see section V.B) and might pose fewer difficulties and risks than methods that rely on an unblinded analysis.

When blinded interim analyses of noninferiority studies are conducted, a larger sample size might improve the statistical power to meet the prospective noninferiority margin and can also increase the potential to demonstrate superiority of the test agent over the comparator in the case where this is true. If the superiority demonstration is also a (secondary) goal of the study sponsor, but the extent of the superiority could not be estimated at the time of study design so that the feasibility of the sample size was uncertain, an adaptive design to modify the study size based on an unblinded interim analysis could be considered. The methods discussed previously are suitable for this adaptive modification if the noninferiority objective is met at the interim analysis point and may call for a statistical adjustment to control the Type I error rate for the superiority comparison.

Many design features of a noninferiority study may not be suitable for adaptation. Chief among these features is the noninferiority margin. The noninferiority margin should be carefully determined during study design, is based largely on historical evidence that does not change, and should not be part of a modification plan for a study. The patient population enrolled in the study may also be difficult to change. The noninferiority margin is based on historical studies that had enrolled patients meeting specified criteria and may apply only to a study population that is similar in important characteristics. Changing the enrolled patient population (e.g., to increase the rate of enrollment) to a population substantially different from that enrolled in the historical studies may compromise the validity of the noninferiority comparison. Similarly, adequate historical data on which to base a noninferiority margin is often available for only one endpoint, so endpoint selection cannot be adaptively modified in the study.

VII.   STATISTICAL CONSIDERATIONS FOR LESS WELL-UNDERSTOOD ADAPTIVE DESIGN METHODS

This section deals with statistical considerations for an adaptive design study that incorporates the more complex approaches described in section VI and that is intended to be an A&WC trial. This section discusses the concern for statistical bias as defined in the ICH E9 guidance. The primary statistical concern of an A&WC study is to control the overall study-wide Type I error rate for all hypotheses tested. This rate can increase in adaptive design studies because of multiplicity related to the multiple adaptation options (and the associated multiple potential hypotheses) or by using biased estimates of the treatment effect. Another concern is avoiding inflation of the Type II error rate (i.e., increased chances of failing to demonstrate a treatment effect when one exists) for the important hypotheses of the study.

A.   Controlling Study-Wide Type I Error Rate

The Type I error rate for the entire study may be increased if inadequate adjustment is made for the many possible choices for adaptation and the many opportunities to demonstrate nominally statistically significant differences. At each stage of interim analysis and adaptation, there can be opportunities for early rejection of some of the several null hypotheses being tested, the possibility of increasing sample sizes, or the selection of the final hypothesis from among several initial hypothesis options. These many choices based on unblinded analyses represent multiplicity that may inflate the Type I error rate that needs to be controlled in A&WC studies.

Avoiding problems with study interpretation and controlling the Type I error rate for all involved hypotheses is best accomplished by prospectively specifying and including in the SAP all possible adaptations that may be considered during the course of the trial. Determining the appropriate statistical correction by taking into account the relative amount of data available at the time of the interim analysis, as well as correlation of the multiple endpoints, is challenging and should be addressed at the protocol design stage. Under some limited circumstances, adaptations not envisioned at the time of protocol design may be feasible, but ensuring control of the Type I error rate remains critical. The flexibility to apply such late changes should be reserved for situations where the change is limited in scope and is particularly important, and should not be proposed repeatedly during a study.

Statistical bias can be introduced into adaptive design studies that make modifications based on interim analyses of a biomarker or an intermediate clinical endpoint thought to be related to the study final endpoint, even though the final study analysis uses a clinical efficacy endpoint. This is because of the correlation between the biomarker and final study endpoint. This potential source of bias should be considered and addressed when the protocol is designed, including appropriate control of the Type I error rate.

One type of adaptation based on an unblinded interim analysis of treatment effects is an increase in the study sample size to maintain study power when the observed effect size is smaller than that initially planned in the protocol. When a statistical bias in the estimate of treatment effect exists, an increase in the sample size does not eliminate the bias. Instead, if flaws in the design (or conduct) of a study introduce a small bias, the increase in sample size can result in the bias increasing the Type I error rate more than would occur without the sample size increase. Thus, the impact of small biases can be magnified when sample size increases are enabled.

B. Statistical Bias in Estimates of Treatment Effect Associated with Study Design

Estimates of the treatment effect are used to make decisions at each stage of an adaptive design study. Because these estimates can be based on a relatively small amount of data, they can be very variable or unstable. The effect estimates for the selected adaptations have the potential to overstate the true effect size because the adaptive choice is usually selected based on the largest of the observed interim treatment effects among the design choice options, which can reflect an unusual distribution of patient observations (often called *random highs* in group sequential designs). This could also lead to selecting a wrong adaptation choice and thus miss detecting a true treatment effect (i.e., lead to a Type II error).

In an adaptive design study, the overall treatment effect is obtained by combining in some manner the treatment effect observed in each stage, and this overall effect estimate should be used for hypothesis testing. How the combining of each stage's data is accomplished can affect the validity of the overall treatment effect estimate. Of particular concern are situations in which the estimates of the treatment effect obtained before and after the design modification differ substantially. Inconsistent treatment effect estimates among the stages of the study can make the overall treatment effect estimate difficult to interpret. The estimate of treatment effect(s) for an adaptive design A&WC study should be critically assessed at the completion of the study.

C. Potential for Increased Type II Error Rate

Adaptive design trials should be planned not only to control the Type I error rate for all involved hypotheses but also to avoid increasing the chance of failing to demonstrate a treatment effect when one exists (the Type II error rate). Type II errors may occur because of suboptimal adaptive selection of design modifications or because of insufficient power to detect a real treatment effect on an endpoint. In general, one of the postulated benefits of adaptive designs is the potential to improve the power of the study to demonstrate a treatment effect through sample size increases or other design modifications.

Adaptive design methods, however, also have the potential to inflate the Type II error rate for one or more hypotheses. An example of this is a study that begins with multiple doses (or populations or other study features) and that early in the study is adaptively modified to eliminate all but one or two doses to be continued to the study's end. This study risks failing to demonstrate treatment effects by making erroneous choices based on interim results that are very variable because of the limited amount of early study data. If this risk is not considered by study planners, an apparently efficient adaptive design study can mislead the drug development program and result in program failure, when it might have succeeded had there been better adaptation choices made. Another example is stopping for futility reasons where a liberal futility stopping criterion may substantially increase the Type II error rate.

D. Role of Clinical Trial Simulation in Adaptive Design Planning and Evaluation

Many of the less well-understood and complex adaptive designs involve several adaptation decision points and many potential adaptations. For study designs that have multiple factors to be simultaneously considered in the adaptive process, it is difficult to assess design performance characteristics and guide sample size planning or optimal design choices because these characteristics might depend upon the adaptations that actually occur. In these cases, trial simulations performed before conducting the study can help evaluate the multiple-trial design options and the clinical scenarios that might occur when the study is actually conducted and can be an important planning tool in assessing the statistical properties of a trial design and the inferential statistics used in the data analysis. section IX provides guidance for the format and content for reporting of clinical trial simulation studies to be included in the adaptive design protocol and the SAP.

In general, clinical trial simulations rely on a statistical model of recognized important design features and other factors, including the posited rate of occurrence of clinical events or endpoint distribution, variability of these factors among patient subsets, postulated relationships between outcomes and prognostic factors, correlation among endpoints, time course of endpoint occurrence or disease progression, and postulated patient withdrawal or dropout patterns, among others. More complex disease models or drug models might attempt to account for changing doses, changing exposure duration, or variability in bioavailability. The multiple ways to adapt and the multiple ways to declare a study as positive can be simulated as part of study planning.

Some modeling and simulation strategies lend themselves to a Bayesian approach that might be useful. The Bayesian framework provides a way to posit models (i.e., priors) for the study design and the adaptive choices as they might probabilistically occur and may aid in evaluating the impact of different assumed distributions for the parameters of the model and modeled sources of uncertainty. The Bayesian approach can be a useful planning tool at the study design stage to accommodate a range of plausible scenarios. Using Bayesian predictive probability, which depends upon probabilities of outcomes conditional on what has been observed up to an interim point in the adaptive study, may aid in deciding which adaptation should be selected, and the study design is still able to maintain statistical control of the Type I error rate in the frequentist design.

Trial simulations can also be helpful in comparing the performance characteristics among several competing designs under different scenarios (e.g., assumptions about drug effect such as the shape and location of the dose–response relationship, magnitude of the response, differing responses in subgroups, distribution of the subgroups in the enrolled population, clinical course of the comparison group [usually the placebo group], and study dropout rate and pattern). The simulations will allow between-design comparisons of the probability of success of the trial for the objective (e.g., to lead to correct dose selection, identify a response above a specific threshold, identify the correct subgroup) and comparisons of the potential size of bias in the treatment effect estimates. For drug development programs where there is little prior experience with the product, drug class, patient population, or other critical characteristics, clinical trial simulations can be performed with a range of potential values for relevant parameters encompassing the uncertainty in current knowledge.

In general, every adaptation may create a new hypothesis whose Type I error rate should be controlled. There have been suggestions that because of the complexity resulting from multiple adaptations and the difficulty in forming an analytical evaluation, modeling and simulation provide a solution for demonstrating control of the Type I error rate for these multiple hypotheses. Using simulations to demonstrate control of the Type I error rate, however, is controversial and not fully understood.

E.   Role of the Prospective Statistical Analysis Plan in Adaptive Design Studies

The importance of prospective specification of study design and analysis is well recognized for conventional study designs, but it is of even greater importance for many of the types of adaptive designs discussed in sections V and VI, particularly where unblinded interim analyses are planned. As a general practice, it is best that adaptive design studies have an SAP that is developed by the time the protocol is finalized. The SAP should specify all of the changes prospectively planned and included in the protocol, describe the statistical methods to implement the adaptations, describe how the analysis of the data from each adaptive stage will be incorporated into the overall study results, and include the justification for the method of control of the Type I error rate and the approach to appropriately estimating treatment effects. The SAP for an adaptive trial is likely to be more detailed and complex than for a nonadaptive trial.

Any design or analysis modification proposed after any unblinded interim analysis raises a concern that access to the unblinded data used in the adaptations may have influenced the decision to implement the specific change selected and thereby raises questions about the study integrity. Therefore, such modifications are generally discouraged. Nonetheless, circumstances can occur that call for the SAP to be updated or for some other flexibility for an unanticipated adaptation. The later in the study these changes or updates are made, the more a concern will arise about the revision's impact. Generally, the justifiable reasons to do so are related to failure of the data to satisfy the statistical assumptions regarding the data (e.g., distribution, proportionality, fit of data to a model).

In general, it is best that any SAP updates occur before any unblinded analyses are performed and that there is unequivocal assurance that the blinding of the personnel determining the modification has not been compromised. A blinded steering committee can make such protocol and SAP changes, as suggested in the ICH E9 guidance and in the DMC guidance, but adaptive designs open the possibility of unintended sharing of unblinded data after the first interim analysis. Any design or analysis modifications made after an unblinded analysis, especially late in the study, may be problematic and should be accompanied by a clear, detailed description of the data firewall between the personnel with access to the unblinded analyses and those personnel making the SAP changes, along with documentation of adherence to these plans. Formal amendments to the protocol and SAP need to be made at the time of such changes (see 1 21 CFR 312.30).

References

Bauer, P. and Köhne, K. 1994. Evaluation of experiments with adaptive interim analyses. *Biometrics*, 50:1029–1041.

Burman, C.-F. and Sonesson, C. 2006. Are flexible designs sound? [With discussion]. *Biometrics*, 62:664–683.

Chin, R., Lee, B.Y. 2008. Principles and Practice of Clinical Trial Medicine. Elsevier,. St. Louis.

Cui, L., Hung, H. M. J. and Wang, S. J. 1999. Modification of sample size in group sequential clinical trials. *Biometrics*. 55: 853: 857.

DeMets, D.L. and Lan, K.K. 1994. Interim analysis: The alpha spending function approach. *Statistics in Medicine*, 13:1341–1352.

Fisher, R. A. 1925. *Statistical methods of research workers*. Oliver and Boyd. Edinburgh.

Fisher, L.D. 1998. *Self-designing clinical trials*. Statistics in Medicine. 17: 1551:1562.

Food and Drug Administration. Guidance for Industry. 2010. Adaptive Design Clinical Trials for Drugs and Biologics.

Hartung, J. and Knapp, G. 2003. A new class of completely self-designing clinical trials. *Biometrical Journal*, 45:3–19.

Lehmann, E.L. 1993. Neyman-Pearson. Theories of Testing Hypothesis. *J. Am. Stat. Assc.* 88: 1242–1249.

Muller, H. H. and Schafer, H. 2001. *Adaptive group sequential designs for clinical trials*. Biometrics. 57: 886–891.

Proschan, M.A. and Hunsberger, S.A. 1995. Designed extension of studies based on conditional power. *Biometrics*, 51:1315–1324.

Tsiatis, A.A. and Mehta, C. 2003. On the inefficiency of the adaptive design for monitoring clinical trials. *Biometrika*, 90:367–378.

Wald, A. 1945. *Sequential Tests of Statistical Hypothesis*. Am Math. Stat. 16:117–186.

4

Specific Requirements for Adaptive Trials[*]

4.1 Requirements for Endpoints in Adaptive Studies

Adaptive studies offer some major advantages compared to traditional trials but in return, they are more difficult to execute and in some cases cannot be used for certain types of trials. Just as dose-ranging trials, as discussed later, lend themselves to adaptive designs, there are some types of trials that are unsuitable for adaptive designs.

One important requirement for adaptive trials is that the endpoint or other data used for the adaptation be available in real time or almost real time. Adaptive trials, by definition, change trial parameters based on data generated during the study. The data that drive the adaptations can be endpoints, variability, dropout rates, or something else, but the time interval between intervention and the data generation must be relatively rapid. Otherwise, the trial may be finished before adaptations can be performed.

Also, most statistical techniques assume a relatively linear relationship between treatment and response. If the relationship is not linear, for example, if doubling the dose quadruples the response and tripling the dose increases response by a factor of 50, then the adaptive technique will need to be modified to account for that.

Drugs that have biphasic effects, delayed response, or rebound can be difficult to evaluate using an adaptive design, although statistical techniques that correct for atypical responses can be used. For example, the time interval between the dose and the outcome can be modified to correct for delayed response. The same is true for drugs with a first dose effect where the response or reaction is the most severe with the first dose, drugs with cumulative dose effect, and drugs with retreatment effects where retreatment after a gap in treatment yields a different response. If the biphasic response, delayed response, or other atypical and nonlinear response is not anticipated or understood, however, the adaptations cannot be properly made and the study may be confounded.

---

[*] Section 4.2 is based on Chin and Lee, 2008, with permission.

In certain types of adaptive designs, such as ones that include crossover or certain intrapatient dose comparisons, the endpoint also needs to be reversible. If it is not reversible, then the carryover effects will confound the subsequent measurements.

Of course, the temporal requirements are dependent on the overall length of the study and the follow-up period. A trial that enrolls in 3 months and has a one-month follow-up period will require data generation within days or weeks of intervention in order to be adaptable. A trial that enrolls in 5 years and has a 10-year follow-up period can be adaptive even with endpoints that take months or years. The key requirement is that the data from one intervention be available rapidly enough so that it can influence the choice of the future intervention in a meaningful fashion.

The most important adaptations are based on endpoints. In that case, if the endpoints become apparent quickly or relatively quickly, then the adaptations can be performed in a straightforward manner. An example of such a response is decrease in pain after administration of an analgesic. The endpoint can be measured in hours or minutes. The measurement can be used to change the next dose in the same patient or in the next patient.

Unfortunately, many clinical endpoints take a long time to manifest. For example, anti-osteoporotic drugs prevent fractures, but the effects may not be apparent for years. With traditional designs, short-term endpoints have of course still been desirable, because they allow shorter studies. However, they have not been essential, because the design is set at the beginning of the study. Therefore, many of the established traditional clinical endpoints such as fractures, mortality, and renal failure take a long time to manifest. They may be poorly suited for adaptive designs where waiting for months may mean that adaptations cannot be performed in a timely manner.

In cases where the effects of the drug are delayed or where the clinical endpoints manifest after a long time, there are several options. First, a surrogate may sometimes be used. For osteoporosis, for example, bone mineral density may be used. Many surrogates can manifest a response long before the clinical endpoint become apparent. Surrogates are discussed in more detail below.

Second, partial data may be used. In many cases, even if the primary endpoint has not been reached, partially complete data may be available. In those cases, with suitable statistical techniques, partial data can be combined with full data and used for the adaptive decisions. For example, in a time-to-event study, even if the event has not yet occurred, partial data can be used for analysis by taking the fact that someone has not had an event yet as a data point. In other words, if a patient has been on a therapy for one month and has not had a flare of a disease, then that is different than if a patient has been on therapy for a year and has not had a flare. If one arm has twice as many patients who have not had a flare, there is usable data that can be used. This takes some statistical manipulation of the data but is readily achievable.

In some studies, the primary endpoint may be a long-term endpoint. In those cases, shorter term endpoints can be used as part of the analysis. For example, if the endpoint is ACR20 response at 12 weeks, the responses at 4 and 8 weeks can be used for the adaptations.

Similarly, components of a composite endpoint can be used for adaptations, if some components respond faster. For example, let's say a study is based on a composite endpoint that includes pain and disability. In that case, pain is likely to respond faster than disability. Therefore, the pain part of the endpoint can be used for the adaptations in those patients who have not been in the study long enough for the disability to be relevant.

Also, for many endpoints that are categorical, such as remission, partial data can be used for analysis. For example, in a macular degeneration study, the proportion of patients with loss of fifteen letters of vision may be the primary endpoint. However, for the adaptations, fewer letters of visual loss or the mean visual loss can be used. For example, patients with five letters of visual loss may be assigned 0.33 points and those with fifteen letters of visual loss be assigned one point. As another example, rather than using ACR20, a finer scale may be needed, such as ACRn, which is a modification that allows construction of ACR0 to ACR100 in 1% increments.

All of these techniques make use of the fact that even before the primary endpoint is reached, there is often partial data about the efficacy that can be used to make better adaptation decisions. However, traditional statistical techniques are not designed to combine complete and incomplete data easily, and you will have to work closely with a statistician to construct appropriate statistical analytic techniques.

Adaptations that rely on dropout rates, variability, or other factors that can be measured continuously can typically be performed without relying on surrogates or other extrapolations.

Please remember that in addition to the above requirements, the design of the trial must be amenable to alteration. If, for example, there is a very long lead time in setting up sites, getting institutional review board approvals, and recruiting patients such that any changes to the study takes 9 months to implement, an adaptive approach may be infeasible.

4.2 Surrogates and Biomarkers

A surrogate endpoint is a measure that fulfills three requirements. First, it correlates with a clinical outcome of interest, usually the primary endpoint in a pivotal study that can qualify for a regulatory approval. Second, it responds to an intervention in a similar fashion as the clinical outcome of interest. It can therefore be used in place of the primary endpoint in many situations. Third, it is in and of itself not the clinical outcome of interest. For example, clearing of infiltrates on a chest x-ray in and of itself does not mean that the patient is doing better.

In contrast, clinical endpoints are endpoints that are in and of themselves meaningful for the patients and physician. Some endpoints that are clinical, as opposed to surrogate, endpoints include death, hospitalization, stroke, and liver failure.

Surrogate endpoints are often used when the final clinical outcome endpoint is not practical or feasible to measure in a clinical trial. It may take too much time, such as development of heart failure in Chagas disease, which can take 30 years. It may occur too infrequently, such as intracranial bleeding with aspirin therapy. It may be too cumbersome to measure, such as actual creatinine clearance rate, which requires invasive infusion and laborious urine collection.

Surrogate endpoints are generally more practical, faster, and/or more numerous than the clinical outcome they replace. For example, blood pressure is a surrogate for stroke. Blood sugar level is a surrogate for renal failure and diabetic retinopathy. Neither blood pressure nor blood sugar levels are in and of themselves clinically significant but are used because of their clinical sequelae. A drug that eliminated the clinical sequelae of hypertension without affecting blood pressure would be just as valuable as one that did both. Other examples of surrogates include x-rays and other radiographic studies for pneumonia and other conditions, guaiac tests, and cardiac ejection fraction.

Outside the clinical trial setting, surrogates are often used to drive clinical practice. Physicians often prescribe antihypertensive drugs to treat high blood pressure, for example, and start antibiotics on the basis of infiltrates on an x-ray. In the context of drug development, however, they are not acceptable for pivotal studies, because more often than not, drugs that have an impressive effect on surrogates end up not having a positive impact on the clinical outcome.

The classic example of this was the cardiac arrhythmia suppression trial (CAST) study. This study was performed because high rates of premature ventricular contractions (PVCs) are predictive of sudden death after myocardial infarction. Based on this, several antiarrhythmic drugs were developed and marketed on the basis of suppression of PVCs. It was taken for granted that these drugs were saving lives, and in fact there was great anguish about the ethics of conducting a placebo-controlled study. Nonetheless, the CAST study was initiated in 1987 comparing flecainide, moricizine, and encainide, which had been shown to be highly effective at reducing PVCs, against placebo. In all, 2,309 patients were randomized.

Because of the expectation that the study would have to be terminated early once the benefit of antiarrhythmic drugs became evident, a data safety monitoring board (DSMB) was included in the study. The DSMB stopped the study early because the patients receiving antiarrhythmic therapy had an unacceptably high mortality. The relative risk (RR) of death and nonfatal events at 10 months was 4.6 in favor of placebo (Cast Investigators 1989).

Since the CAST study, numerous other surrogate endpoints, including even blood pressure and blood sugar levels, have been shown instances not to predict clinical outcome. In general, surrogate endpoints should be used only when a clinical endpoint is not feasible. A surrogate endpoint is never as informative or clinically relevant as the clinical endpoint. Moreover, a surrogate endpoint that works for one drug may not for another drug with a different mechanism of action, even for the same disease. As a result, regulatory authorities and many clinicians insist on clinical rather than surrogate endpoints.

Many measurements that correlate with disease do not correlate with response to therapy. For example, *Helicobacter pylori* antibody may correlate with the likelihood of developing duodenal ulcers. But antibiotic treatment that eradicates the infection will not reverse a patient's antibody-positive status. The antibody is a good diagnostic biomarker but not a good surrogate.

A good surrogate must be in the causal pathway. This is illustrated in Figure 4.1.

Fully validated surrogate endpoints are rare. Validated surrogates are surrogate endpoints for which it has been shown that drugs that affected the surrogate also affected the clinical endpoint and that drugs that did not affect the surrogate failed to show a clinical effect. Also, ideally the validation should be based on drugs similar to the new drug that you want to study because a surrogate that is valid for one type of drug that acts on one part of the biological process may not be valid for a different type of drug that acts on a different part.

4.3 Practical Requirements

In addition to the above, there are practical requirement for an adaptive study, some of which have been previously discussed. First, the adaptation must be practicable. For example, if the institutional review boards take too long to approve adaptations, if the regulators do not approve the adaptations, or if the turnaround for measuring the pharmacokinetic marker being used for the adaptation is too long, adaptive designs cannot be used. In addition, in situations such as very remote areas such as parts of Africa, where paper-based systems must be used rather than electronic data capture and transportation of supplies and drugs take weeks or months, adaptive designs are not appropriate.

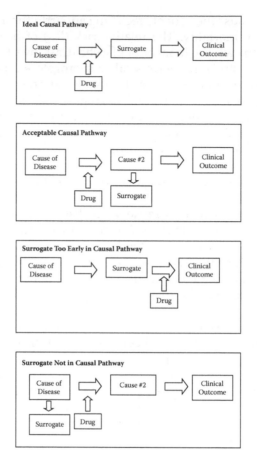

FIGURE 4.1
Surrogate endpoints and the causal pathway. (Reprinted from Chin and Lee. 2008. With permission.)

References

CAST Investigators. 1989. Preliminary report. NEJM. 321:406–412.
Chin, R. and Lee, B.Y. 2008. *Principles and Practice of Clinical Trial Medicine*. Elsevier: St. Louis, MO.

5

Adaptive Randomization and Allocation[*]

5.1 Traditional Fixed Allocation

In conventional studies, the allocation methodology is determined at the beginning. These schemes are called *fixed* or *static allocation*. In adaptive clinical trials, on the other hand, allocation rules can change over the course of the study. In other words, adaptive randomization or dynamic allocation can be used. In this section, types of randomizations will be reviewed, starting with traditional randomization and then exploring various adaptive randomization schemes.

There are several ways of allocating or assigning patients to treatments, but randomization is the most common. *Randomization* is the process of randomly assigning subjects to different study arms. Other allocation methods include assignment based on nonrandomization such as assigning every other patient to the treatment arm.

Randomization helps accomplish several objectives. It produces groups that are balanced for both known and unknown risk factors and covariates. It is impossible to match patients in each arm on each of the infinite number of variables that might affect the course of disease and likelihood of response. Randomization, if the sample size is adequate, ensures that the treatment and control groups are adequately balanced with regard to baseline characteristics, including unmeasured or unknown characteristics.

Without randomization, the investigator may select patients for particular therapy based on prognosis or other characteristics that might impact outcome.

In the past, randomization codes were generated in advance and a statistician kept the codes and allocated them manually one by one as the need arose in the course of the study, but today, most randomization codes are generated on demand by a computer.

Of note, if the adaptation changes the demographics of the groups so that there is an imbalance between the groups, that can introduce bias. Standard randomization usually does not cause this difficulty, but adaptive randomization algorithms that take into account both demographics and responses can pose this danger, as discussed later.

[*] Parts of this chapter are based on Chin and Lee, 2008. With permission.

The ratio of randomization is the proportion of patients assigned to the arms relative to the other arms. The most common randomization ratio in clinical trials is 1:1, which maximizes statistical power for nonadaptive studies. A 1:1 randomization ratio means that equal numbers of patients will be randomized into each of the two study arms.

Using an unequal ratio such as 2:1 can allocate more patients to receive the active study intervention than placebo, affording patients a greater chance of receiving a potential active treatment. This can yield benefit to the patient and increase enrollment rates. Unequal ratios decrease power of the study.

There are several different types of randomization as detailed below. Although regulators sometimes take a dim view of adaptive randomization, some traditional randomization methodologies have long incorporated adaptive elements.

5.2 Simple Randomization

Simple randomization is the most straightforward method of random assignment. Each patient has a fixed probability of being assigned to each study arm. In equal allocations, each subject has an equal probability of being assigned to each of the study arms. In unequal or weighted allocations, patients are more likely to end up in certain study arms than others but the probability is set at the beginning of the study and does not change.

Pure simple randomizations are not adaptive. If the randomization generator is programmed so that the randomization is truly random, it is a nonadaptive randomization. This sort of pure randomization poses the risk that one arm may end up enrolling more patients than another, because the number of patients in each arm is truly random. For larger studies, minor disparity in the number of arms in each arm will not be a major problem but for smaller studies it may be.

Therefore, most randomization that is considered to be simple randomization is actually restricted randomization. The randomization generator is programmed to balance the total number of patients enrolled into the arms. Restricted randomization is explained below, and it is an adaptive randomization.

5.3 Restricted and Blocked Randomization

In relatively small studies, simple randomization may result in unbalanced groups. For example, if you had only twenty patients for a study and two study arms, there is reasonably high probability that one arm could have twelve patients and the other would have eight. Moreover, there may be a temporal imbalance in study group assignment. More patients early on in the study may end up in one particular arm and late in the study in the other arm. This can increase the risk of temporal bias. For example, if a study of flu infections is performed, and more patients are enrolled into arm one at the beginning and less at the end, the drift of the flu genotypes over time may introduce a bias.

Restricted randomization limits the number of patients that can be randomized to a particular arm. So for example, if in a 100-patient study, 50 patients have been enrolled into arm A and 40 into arm B, the next 10 patients would be randomized to arm B.

Blocked randomization is a subset of restricted randomization and is similar, except instead of waiting until the end of the study, the randomization scheme balances the randomization across the arms more frequently. In block randomization, each set of patients is allocated a randomization such that at the end of each block, the number of patients in each arm is balanced. For example, it might balance the randomization every ten patients. This makes temporal bias less likely because at every tenth patient the arms will be balanced across the groups.

Small block sizes smaller than six patients should be avoided in small studies. The smaller the block size, the easier it will be for investigators to guess the study group assignments.

Restricted and block randomizations are really a type of adaptive randomization.

Because the probability of being randomized to a particular arm is dependent on the previous randomization of the patients, they represent a form of adaptive randomization although it is not traditionally recognized as such. In other words, the probability of any patient being assigned to a particular arm is dependent on the randomization of the previous patients.

This is true even if the allocation codes and blocks are predetermined at the beginning of the study, because the randomization of the patient is influenced by the order of the patients enrolled into the study, and therefore the likelihood of being enrolled into a particular arm is adaptive. Similarly, allocation schemes that alternate between arms in a fixed pattern are adaptive.

5.4 Stratified, Nested, and Similar Randomization

Stratified randomization classifies patients into strata based on one or more baseline characteristics and the randomization is performed independently for each strata. The strata may be based on a variety of factors such as sex, age, study site, disease severity, disease subtype, and concomitant medications.

Stratified randomization can be helpful when certain baseline characteristics are expected to influence the outcome of interest. For instance, anterior myocardial infarction patients fare worse than those with inferior myocardial infarctions. So, if 50% of the myocardial infarctions in study arm A are anterior and 20% of the myocardial infarctions in study arm B are anterior, study arm A is likely to have a higher mortality regardless of the intervention. In a very large trial, most baseline characteristics will be naturally balanced across the different study arms, but small trials run the risk that one or more characteristic will be unbalanced.

Stratified randomization helps make each of the individual subgroups more homogenous, which can aid subsequent analysis and may increase the power of the study. Moreover, conclusions specific to the strata can be made with more certainty because the strata were identified and randomized separately. However, there are limits to how many strata you can employ, because with a lot of strata, each stratum would have very few patients. Stratification can be logistically challenging as well.

Pure stratified randomizations are not adaptive if the stratification is based on patient baseline characteristics, because the baseline characteristics are not data generated in the course of the study.

Related to stratified randomization are fixed allocations. This method allocates based on a fixed characteristic that is patient dependent, such as the last digit of the social security number. For example, patients with an odd social security number receive a placebo and those with an even number receive drug. This type of randomization is not adaptive either.

Nested randomizations in which sites or other blocks are randomized and then the patients are subrandomized are not adaptive unless block randomization is used.

5.5 Balancing (Covariate) Adaptive Randomization

Covariate adaptive randomization maintains a balance of relevant characteristics among the different study arms over the course of the study. During a trial, the distribution of covariates such as age, sex, or comorbid conditions may become unbalanced between the arms. Covariate adaptive randomization changes the likelihood of the arm that the patients will be assigned based on how many patients with certain covariates have been enrolled into each arm. Of course, this can only be done with covariates that are measured.

An optimal design approach uses a treatment estimator—essentially a score calculated on the basis of multiple patient factors—and adapts the randomization to equalize the scores of the patients assigned to each arm.

There are specific techniques for covariate randomization, such as Urn randomization and Efron's weighted coin, both of which change the likelihood of randomization into the arms based on the imbalances to date (Efron 1971). Urn's technique changes the likelihood of randomization into the groups after each time a patient is randomized (Wei 1988). After a patient has been randomized into one arm, the randomization algorithm is changed to account for the latest patient's covariates and randomization. Efron's technique allocates the probability based on the distribution of imbalance in the covariates before each randomization.

Covariate adaptive randomization is adaptive randomization, as the name suggests. Performed properly, it should pose minimal statistical risk, because it should not normally introduce a bias. However, some theoretical risk has been postulated. For example, adjusting randomization for known covariates may potentially introduce bias from unknown covariates. However, this is largely a theoretical concern that would be found very rarely and only when the covariates have systematic correlation with an unknown covariate.

One danger of covariate adjusted randomization is temporal effects. Some patient characteristics, external factors, and/or responses may change. Covariate-adjusted characteristics (e.g., blood pressure, heart rate, comorbid conditions) may fluctuate during the course of the study. The characteristics initially may seem unbalanced but over the course of time actually be balanced or vice versa.

5.6 Response (Outcome) Adaptive Randomization

Response adaptive randomization changes the randomization scheme based on response to therapy. For example, if patients in arm A exhibit a better response than patients in arm B, then the likelihood of randomization into arm A can be increased.

This method can increase the likelihood of subsequent patients being assigned to effective treatment groups. To utilize response adaptive randomization, treatment responses need to be relatively rapid and easily measurable. Studies with drugs that exert effects slowly are poorly suited for response adaptive randomizations or to adaptive trial design for that matter unless a biomarker or surrogate is available.

There are several variants of response adaptive design. A common technique is the "play the winner design," of which there are several subvariants. With this technique, when a patient experiences a response in one arm, the likelihood of subsequent patients being randomized to that arm is increased. Conversely, if a patient fails therapy, then the likelihood of patients being randomized to that arm is decreased.

The utility model design always randomizes patients to the group that has the highest response rate. The utility offset model design randomizes patients to groups in proportion to the relative benefit observed in each arm.

In other words, if arm A has demonstrated twice the response rate as arm C, then the likelihood of being randomized to arm A would be twice as great as the likelihood of getting randomized to arm C.

In another variant, if a patient exhibits a response, then the next patient always gets randomized to that arm, and randomization is switched only (and always) in case of failure.

A "drop the loser" design eliminates the entire arm when the arm appears to not be working.

A doubly adaptive biased coins design uses the equivalent of a coin flip to randomize patients but weights the coin flip based on both the previous assignments of the patients and responses of the different study groups.

One potential problem with adaptive randomization is potential temporal effects. Response to treatment can oscillate over time. Patients may respond to a treatment early on but later become unresponsive or vice versa.

Response adaptive randomization is adaptive. Done properly, this technique should not introduce a bias and therefore it should not increase statistical risk. The issue, of course, with this technique is that with many drugs, higher efficacy is seen at higher doses and the higher doses often have worse safety profiles. Though it is a reasonable goal to maximize the number of patients in the efficacious arms, this scheme may be neither the safest nor the most powerful from a statistical analysis viewpoint.

5.7 Combination and Multimodal Randomization

Variations on the above randomizations are possible, such as randomization based on both covariates and previous assignment; based on both responses and previous assignments; or based on covariates, response, and previous assignments.

One example would be to assess biomarker status (covariate) and response to therapy and enrich the patients with the covariate into the arms more likely to show a benefit. There is significant risk of interactions in such schemes. Specifically, there is a danger that by using both covariates and outcome, the randomization will enrich the treatment arm with patients who are less sick or otherwise have different prognostic factors than the untreated arm.

The adaptations in randomizations can be applied in two different scales. One option is on a patient-by-patient basis. After each patient is enrolled, the adaptation scheme is updated. Alternatively, the randomization scheme can be updated after multiple patients have been randomized. For example, it can be updated after a prespecified number of patients—let's say ten patients or twenty patients, for example—have been randomized or based on changes that occur after certain cohorts of patients have been enrolled. Alternatively, the randomization scheme can be updated once the imbalance—covariate, response, or otherwise—reaches a certain level.

5.8 Bayesian Randomization

Although adaptive randomization is generally performed with standard statistical techniques, one or more of the above factors can be combined to allow Bayesian randomization. With this technique, the information from prior patients is combined to produce a posterior probability that is used to influence randomizations of future patients. The patients are randomized preferentially into arms that appear to have the best efficacy, best suited to insure equal distribution of covariates, etc.

5.9 Adaptation of Inclusion and Exclusion Criteria Based on Blinded Data

One relatively uncontroversial adaptive design is prespecified adaptation of inclusion and exclusion criteria to shift the enrollment in one direction or another. For example, if a prespecified distribution, say, of 60% inferior myocardial infarction patients and 40% anterior myocardial infarction patients, is desirable for a study, then a prespecified change in the inclusion criteria to favor patients with greater or less ST segment elevation might be used. Alternatively, the protocol might specify that certain criteria could be modified after examining the screening logs for screen failures to insure target enrollment distributions.

In practice, this type of adaptation is not used very often because a simpler way of achieving similar results is to stratify the patients and to specify the number of patients in each strata or simply to limit the number of patients in specific subgroups.

Slightly more useful are strategies to examine a subgroup at the interim analysis and to drop a subgroup. With this technique, all patients who have been enrolled into that subgroup to date would be dropped from the final analysis and no further patients would be enrolled into the subgroup.

One way to implement this statistically is to have a certain amount of alpha allocated to a null hypothesis for the subgroup or to a null hypothesis comparing the subgroup to the other subgroup(s). However, both of these methods would spend alpha.

Alternatively, the subgroups could be dropped on the basis of unblinded data such as variance within the particular group or event rate in the control arm of the subgroup. For instance, if it is not known what the basal event rate is in a subgroup, an interim analysis can be performed in which the rule is that if the event rate is very low, the subgroup can be dropped. This would remove a subgroup that would otherwise dilute the power of the study because the subgroup would lower the overall event rate. This would not require spending of alpha.

However, the common practice of broadening the inclusion criteria because of slow enrollment is not adaptive. If performed solely for the purposes of increasing the enrollment rate, and in an unplanned fashion—that is, the enrollment rate was poorly estimated at the beginning of the trial—this would be an instance not of an adaptive trial but rather poor trial planning.

5.10 Patient Enrichment Adaptations

One adaptive trial element that has been used for many years is enrichment of patient populations. One example is the run-in period. A run-in period occurs before randomization and gives patients an opportunity to wean off other medications or to be initiated on the study drug, among other things. A run-in period is adaptive in that the patient population enrolled in the study can be changed by events that occur in the study, albeit before the patients are randomized.

A run-in period can accomplish many objectives, including the following:

- Exclude patients who do not tolerate the intervention.
- Screen out noncompliant patients.
- Screen out placebo responders.
- Screen for intervention response. Sometimes identifying those patients most likely to respond to the intervention is necessary. For example, knowing the response can affect study arm assignment (e.g., you may want a balance of different responses in different study arms).
- Establish dosing and other intervention parameters. During a run-in period, you can "tinker with" and adjust different intervention parameters (e.g., dose size, dose frequency, medical device setting, or medical device positioning).

Elements in the run-in period that result in patients being excluded from the study should be considered to be adaptive. Of course, employing run-in periods can introduce some problems:

- During a run-in period, patients' characteristics (e.g., disease severity, weight, or lab values) may change so that they are no longer eligible for the trial.
- Patients may suffer disease progression or flares while off their usual medications.
- Run-in periods require time, effort, and resources that may otherwise be used for the study periods.
- Excluding nonresponders, placebo responders, or noncompliant patients may make the study less applicable to the real-world population.

A screening period is also similar to the run-in period but often is considered distinct from it because patients are typically not officially enrolled into the study for the screening period. It is a period that allows time for the logistics of performing the tests (e.g., if an oncology trial requires histological confirmation of the tumor type as part of the inclusion criteria, then the time spent waiting for the central laboratory to read and prepare the report is part of the screening period).

References

Chin, R. and Lee, B.Y. 2008. *Principles and Practice of clinical trial medicine*. Elsevier: St. Louis, MO.

Efron, B. 1971. *Forcing a sequential experiment to be balanced*. Biometrika. 58: 403–417.

Wei, L. J. and Lachin, J. M. 1988. *Properties of the Urn Randomization in Clinical Trials*. Cont. Clin. Trials. 9: 345–364.

6

Sample Size Reestimation

6.1 Background

One of the recurring challenges in clinical study design is proper sample size estimation. Often, the information necessary for determining the sample size is not available or poorly reliable. For example, the variance for an outcome endpoint, such as ACR20 reduction, may not be well described for the population of interest. The information may not be reliable because there is an insufficient number of studies, the studies were different in some way from the new study, or the execution of the studies were poor.

Underpowered studies can result in Type II error or false-negative results. Overpowered studies can also be unnecessarily expensive and may expose more patients needlessly to an ineffective therapy or placebo. Improper sample size estimation may also lead to drugs never being developed because it is believed falsely that the study would be too large. It is therefore important to have a reliable estimate of the variance or a way of designing a study so that it can be changed if the variance or other estimates turn out to be inaccurate.

Factors that determine sample size include event rate in the control group, variance in the outcome variable, expected effect size, and dropout rate. Many of these parameters can be used to estimate and to adjust the sample size, either in a blinded or unblinded fashion.

Adaptive study designs offer a method for changing the sample size of the study during the course of the study. This is called *sample size reestimation*. Of the sample size reestimation techniques, there are several different categories, each with a varying degree of flexibility.

A fixed sample size reestimation method uses a prespecified, fixed, and usually identical sample size per stage. Information-based sample size reestimation changes the sample size based on the goal of keeping the amount of information in each stage fixed. An error spending approach changes the sample size in a flexible manner, but the information used in each stage is independent of information in the different stages (Lan 1983). Sequentially planned decision procedure bases sample sizes going forward on an integrated test statistic that is calculated on the cumulative information to date

(Schmitz 1993). The most flexible technique relies on unblinded data on the actual treatment effect and is a function of conditional power. These are described in more detail below.

6.2 Sample Size Reestimation Based on Blinded Data

Several well-accepted techniques exist for revising study sample sizes based on blinded data. Several parameters that can impact sample size can be determined during the course of a study without resorting to unblinding. These include variance of particular variables, length of survival, mean effect size, and several other factors. Sample sizes can be changed based on prespecified rules, if the initial estimates for these factors are not borne out by the study.

For example, if the initial sample size was based on a variance of two-point change in the expanded disability status scale (EDSS) score for a treatment for multiple sclerosis, and the actual variance turns out to be one, the sample size can be decreased. Sample size reestimation based on the variance is the most common type of blinded sample size reestimation.

If the parameter is a so-called nuisance parameter—a parameter such as variance or other factors that do not have a relationship to the endpoint and therefore do not give an indication as to whether the therapy is efficacious— there is little or no statistical risk. The statistical validity of the final analysis is generally preserved because the nuisance parameter does not affect or unblind the magnitude of treatment effect. It should be noted, however, that with each sample size reestimation performed, there is potential sacrifice of some statistical power.

Also, if the sample size is adjusted because of a safety endpoint unrelated to the primary efficacy endpoint, there is little statistical risk. For example, the high-dose arm of a trial may be discontinued because of excess adverse events, but that would not affect the statistical rigor of the study, because the safety endpoint should be unrelated to the primary endpoint, nor should it require unblinding of the primary endpoint.

A more difficult situation arises if an efficacy endpoint is used for sample size reestimation but that particular endpoint is not the primary endpoint. For example, in a rheumatoid arthritis study, joint erosion might be the primary endpoint. Let's say that the sample size is adjusted based on ACR20 scores. There is often a correlation between joint erosion and ACR20. Although a case could be made that examining the ACR20 data does not necessarily unblind the joint erosion endpoint, the magnitude of ACR20 can indicate the degree of treatment effect for joint erosion. The conservative approach would be to treat such sample size reestimation as one based on unblinded data.

If subgroups of particular interest have been stratified in order to draw conclusions about the subgroups, and the variance or other factors that impact sample size is contrary to initial estimates, the sample sizes can be changed.

For time-to-event studies, the sample size may be based not on the total enrollment but on the total number of outcome events. This type of sample size determination is sometimes not recognized to be adaptive design. Strictly speaking, this is an archetypical example of adaptive design because the sample size reestimation is essentially built into the protocol and enrollment termination. It is an example of automatic sample size reestimation.

6.3 Sample Size Reestimation Based on Unblinded Data

Sample size reestimation can also be based on unblinded data, including the size of the drug effect that is observed at the interim analysis. However, sample size reestimation based on unblinded data carries more risk from a statistical and operational viewpoint. Of course, the unblinded data can be very informative for adjusting the sample size. Most or all of the sample size reestimation based on unblinded data is based on the *p* value combination theories of Bauer (1994).

One technique, described by Fisher (1998) and mentioned earlier, is called a *variance-spending method* or *self-designing method* (also called an *error spending approach*). This method allows the sample size and the proportion of the test statistic's variance to be determined sequentially for each stage or even after each patient in a trial based on data available at the time of the decision. All data can be used for the final analysis, including data about the outcome, by combining the *p* values as explained in Chapter 3.

Essentially, this technique divides the study into very small steps and sequentially allocates alpha at each step. After each step, which can be after any number of patients, the amount of alpha to be spent in the next step is determined via an algorithm. The alpha is then used to change the sample size. This technique allows use of unblinded data. The technique can be used for adaptation of parameters other than sample sizes as well.

Proschan and Hunsberger (1995) described the other main technique for unblinded sample size reestimation. They introduced a technique for using a conditional error function, which defines how many additional patients should be enrolled after the interim analysis. The conditional error function is prespecified at the beginning of the study and, based on the unblinded look at the effect size, the additional number of patients specified by the error function is enrolled. This concept is a bit abstract, but the function just means that you prespecify how many more patients you will enroll given a certain result at the interim analysis. The data from both stages can then be combined for the final analysis.

Information-based sample size calculation or reestimation is a way of specifying the size of the study not by sample size or by the number of events but by specifying the amount of information gathered (Mehta and Tsiatis 2001). The information is typically a statistical parameter. This parameter might be made up, for example, of the mean response rate in the study arms and the difference in the rates and the standard error. Basically, you can specify that the study will continue until it has sufficient power to determine whether the drug works or not.

The above techniques usually require using unblinded data, often multiple times. It therefore requires interim analysis. It is also logistically challenging, because at the beginning of the study, it is not clear how big the sample size will be. The initial sample size must be based on assumptions, just like a traditional study.

In some cases, reestimation based on unblinded data does not impact statistical power. These are reestimation based on safety or other parameters that are independent of the primary efficacy endpoint. For example, if estimation of a rare adverse event is one of the secondary endpoints and the unblinded analysis indicates that the rate is too low and the sample size needs to be increased, that could be done without affecting the power for the primary efficacy endpoint. In some cases, designs that only change the sample size based on the unblinded variability data and do not allow for other changes or termination of the study at the interim analysis do not require spending any alpha at the interim analysis.

6.4 Adjustment in Follow-Up Time

In some cases, rather than increasing the sample size of patients, the length of follow-up or the number of events that will be collected is adapted. Typically, this presents the same benefits and risks as the adjustments in sample size.

6.5 Internal Pilot Studies

Sometimes, the initial stage of an adaptive or multistage study is called an *internal pilot study*. If the results of the pilot study will not be used as part of the final analysis for the study, the pilot study may be considered to be a separate study and not part of an adaptive design. It is only if the results of the pilot stage are intended to be combined with the results from a later stage in the final analysis and hypothesis testing that the pilot study should be considered to be part of an adaptive study.

6.6 Additional Rules

It is possible to put boundaries on allowable sample size adaptations. In cases where a minimum size of one of the arms is prespecified, this is called a *restricted sampling rule.*

Information-based design, unlike traditional designs, does not make the sample sizes fixed in advance but rather bases the sample sizes on the amount of information accumulated during the study.

An error spending approach offers a great deal of flexibility in sample sizes, and the sample sizes can be different from stage to stage because the amount of alpha spent is different in each stage of the study. Sequential decision procedures based on the current value of the test statistic allow future samples sizes to be a function of the test statistic.

The most flexible sample size reestimation uses an estimated treatment effect to calculate conditional power to change the sample size. *Conditional power* is the power to achieve a positive study result based on the data collected up to the interim and based on the original specified treatment effect. In other words, it is the likelihood that the study is large enough to show a difference if the difference exists. It is not the power to show a difference if the treatment effect seen at the interim analysis continues to be the treatment effect through the end of the study.

Some sample size reestimation techniques use the treatment effect seen at the interim analysis (rather than the treatment effect assumptions from the beginning of the study) to resize the study, but this can be risky because the treatment effect seen at the interim analysis can vary widely. This is because the number of patients at the interim analysis may be quite small. Basing the sample size on the treatment effect from the interim analysis therefore can lead to unnecessarily large sample sizes. It may be better to base the sample size reestimation on the original treatment effect, taking into account the variance and the conditional power. This can avoid mistakes in estimating the new sample size.

References

Bauer, P. and Kohne, K. 1994. Evaluation of experiments with adaptive interim analyses. Biometrics. 50: 1029–1041.

Fisher, L.D. 1998. Self-designing clinical trials. *Statistics in Medicine*, 17:1551–1562.

Lan, K.K.G. and DeMets, D.L. 1983. Discrete sequential boundaries for clinical trials. *Biometrika*, 70:659–663.

Mehta, C.R. and Tsiatis, A.A. 2001. Flexible sample size considerations using information-based interim monitoring. *Drug Information Journal*, 35:1095–1112.

Proschan, M. A. and Hunsberger, S.A. 1995. *Designed extension of studies based on conditional power*. Biometrics. 51: 1315–1324.

Schmitz, N. 1993. Optimal Sequentially Planned Decision Procedures. *Lecture Notes in Statistics*, 79.

7

Traditional Dosing

7.1 Introduction

Adaptive design is frequently used in dose finding studies, for reasons that will be delineated in the next section. However, in order to understand the impact that adaptive designs have on dosing, it is important to understand the traditional goals and techniques as they relate to dosing.

Most clinical studies involve an intervention such as a drug, a medical device, or surgery, because the aim of most trials is to assess the effectiveness and safety of an intervention. This intervention can be therapeutic or preventive; invasive or noninvasive; acute or chronic. For this book, we mainly discuss drugs but many of the principles can also apply to other therapeutics.

For an intervention meant to be studied in a clinical trial, the intervention must meet several requirements. First, it must be reproducible and standardizable. An intervention that cannot be standardized, such as a difficult surgical technique that is performed differently by each surgeon, cannot be properly studied in a clinical trial. Similarly, for a drug, each pill must contain the same amount and form of the drug. This is not always trivial at the early stages of drug development, especially for biologics and vaccines.

If a drug must be mixed by the pharmacist or administered on a weight-based dosing or must be delivered over a specified time course, the target dosing may not correspond to actual dosing. If the drug is improperly stored, the potency may be affected. Once again, this is a problem more common in early clinical trials. Also, it must be clear when the intervention begins and ends. This is not difficult for most drugs but is difficult for other types of interventions such as exercise regimens.

It is important to keep patient safety paramount in all stages of clinical development, but this is particularly true during Phase I, where the risk is the greatest and information is the most limited. Administering an intervention to patients before much is known about its safety is an inherently risky endeavor. All dose-ranging trials should proceed carefully and cease before patients are subject to significant harm. You should never escalate to a higher dose until you have collected enough data and are convinced that escalation is justified and poses acceptable risk.

117

Choosing a target dose can be very subjective and challenging. Different physicians and different regulatory agencies can look at the same set of data and derive different target doses. Also, depending on the severity of the disease and the available alternatives, the risk–benefit ratio may make sense in one circumstance and not in another.

7.2 Definitions and Objectives of Dose Selection

Dose selection, exploration, and characterization are three key components of dosing. Dose selection is deciding which doses to test on a group of patients. Dose exploration involves testing the different doses and observing their effects and safety. Dose exploration leads to dose characterization, the description of the relationships between the dose and clinical (and nonclinical) effects.

The overall goal of dose selection, exploration, and characterization is not just to identify doses that are safe and effective but also to paint a comprehensive picture of the following:

- Relationships between dose and efficacy, safety, and convenience.
- Parameters that affect these relationships.
- Dosing regimens that appropriately balance efficacy and safety.

You will want a full understanding of how different doses behave in a wide variety of situations, such as the distribution of efficacy and toxicity in the population and whether the patients experiencing the adverse events are the ones exhibiting response. Being able to predict (if possible) which patients will respond and which will suffer toxicity would allow clinicians to select the right doses and appropriate measures to avoid or alleviate adverse effects.

In clinical practice, clinicians often use doses that are different from that indicated on the label. There are many reasons for this. The patient may be of a different height, weight, ethnicity, age, or gender from those studied in the clinical trial. The patient's comorbid conditions, concomitant medications, and relevant physiologic parameters also may be unlike those in the clinical trial population. The same toxicity may be more or less problematic to different patients (e.g., losing sensation in the fingers may be more significant for a surgeon than an accountant). Or a patient may not be able to pay for a full dose. The patient may have a terminal disease and have no other option, prompting the clinician to try higher and riskier doses.

A dose–response curve is a graph that plots the dose (or the logarithm of the dose) on the x-axis and the response on the y-axis. The maximal tolerated dose is the highest dose that will not cause any harm or, in some indications such as oncology, the highest dose with acceptable toxicity levels.

From the efficacy and safety parameters, you can calculate the therapeutic index (also known as *therapeutic ratio* or *margin of safety*). This is the ratio of the dose that causes toxic effects divided by the dose that generates the desired therapeutic effects.

7.3 Issues

There are a number of challenges in dose selection. The first is risk–benefit ratio optimization. Risk–benefit ratio optimization refers to the process of defining what doses maximize the benefits of the intervention while minimizing the dangers. All drugs have toxicity at high doses, so completely eliminating risk is impossible. And higher doses tend to be more effective. So, the challenge is to find the appropriate balance between benefits and risks.

Unfortunately, risk–benefit ratio optimization is rarely the same for all patients because they and their underlying diseases are very heterogeneous (e.g., different metabolism, body sizes, rates of exercise, exposure to sunlight, compliance, genders, ages, concomitant medications, races, and tolerance levels). Different patients may respond to a given dose in different ways. Some will improve more and faster. Some will suffer worse or more frequent side effects. In general, the more heterogeneous the response, the more difficult it is to find acceptable balance of safety and efficacy.

This highlights the second challenge in dose selection: heterogeneity management. Heterogeneity makes assessing the risk–benefit ratio complicated. Simply calculating the mean or median risk–benefit ratio for each dose may not be enough, because the risk–benefit ratio may differ for different patients. Characterizing the risk–benefit ratio distribution for each dose as much as possible should be the goal. Ideally, you should be able to generate a histogram of risk–benefit ratios for each tested dose and identify such parameters as the 10th and 90th percentile. Moreover, quantifying the risks and benefits can be problematic. Is a moderate response equal to half of a full response? Clinical trials are good at generating population-level dosing data, but you then must use these data to determine doses for individual patients.

When significant heterogeneity exists, you may have to use any number of methods to make heterogeneous responses more homogeneous. Adaptive design offers one solution, but other methods are as follows:

- Individualizing Doses: Individualization of doses is the most common method and involves varying the dose by a parameter that drives heterogeneity (e.g., if you find that drug response varies by patient weight, you may have to give heavier patients higher doses than lighter patients).

- Titrating to an Endpoint: An alternative method is choosing a relevant clinical endpoint (i.e., outcome) and adjusting the dose for each patient until the endpoint reaches a certain value (e.g., changing the medication dose until a certain blood pressure is achieved).

- Dosing by Subpopulation: Another method is to identify subpopulations that may respond differently to the drug and giving each subpopulation a different appropriate dose (e.g., men may receive higher doses than women or African Americans may require different doses than Latinos; patients with liver failure may only tolerate lower doses). In some cases, the drug may not be indicated or safe for certain subpopulations.

The third factor in dose selection is that frequency of dosing must be balanced with dosing. For example, for radiation therapy, fractionating the dose into multiple smaller doses may reduce toxicity.

The fourth factor is that dose–response may not be static. There may be a cumulative effect, where the response increases with increasing doses, or attenuation/tolerance, where the opposite happens. With some drugs, there is rebound, where the body builds up an opposite reaction to the drug and when the drug is discontinued, the opposite pharmacological effect to the effect of the drug occurs. For example, when beta blockers are discontinued, heart rate often will rebound and become even faster than it was at baseline before administration of the beta blocker.

Some drugs also exhibit a delayed effect, such that the effect of the drug is not apparent immediately. If an effect of a drug extends into another dosing period, this is called a carryover effect. A washout period may be necessary, during which time the drug and its effects dissipate from the body. Similarly, there might be different response with fed/fasted state, time of day, and various other factors, not to mention differences caused by sex, renal clearance, and hepatic clearance. All of these factors must be considered when dose–response relationship is being elucidated.

7.4 Pharmacokinetics

Extensive discussion of pharmacokinetics and pharmacodynamics is beyond the scope of this book, but key concepts will be briefly summarized. Pharmacokinetics (PK) is the study of the way drugs are absorbed, distributed, metabolized, and eliminated by the body. Pharmacodynamics (PD) is the study of the action of a drug on the body over a period of time. PK looks at what the body does to a drug, and PD looks at what a drug does to the body.

There are five steps in the passage of a drug through the human body:

1. Administration: You give the patient the drug through one of a variety of possible routes, such as oral, intravenous, intramuscular, and subcutaneously.

2. Absorption: The drug moves from where it is administered into systemic circulation.

3. Distribution: The drug spreads throughout the body.

4. Metabolism: The body alters the chemical structure of the drug.

5. Elimination: The drug is excreted from the body.

There are several common measures of bioavailability: the maximum (peak) plasma drug concentration, the time at which this peak occurs (peak time), and the area under the plasma concentration–time curve (AUC). More important than bioavailability or blood level of the drug is the concentration of the drug that reaches the target tissue and cells, but this is often very difficult to measure.

Peak plasma drug concentration informs you about the extent of absorption (the greater the absorption, the higher the peak); peak time tells you about absorption rate (slowing absorption delays the peak time); the AUC provides information about both extent and rate. The AUC reveals the total amount of drug that reaches systemic circulation.

In the bloodstream, a percentage of the total drug amount is bound to blood proteins (e.g., albumin, lipoproteins, or hemoglobin).

Several factors can affect bioavailability, including physiochemical properties of the drug such as solubility, concomitant food, and concomitant diseases such as gasteroenteritis.

Only unbound drug can move out of the blood into the tissue to exert its effects. So it is often useful to calculate the percentage or fraction of unbound drug. Many biologics cause some degree of antibody formation. For example, infliximab causes anti-infliximab antibodies in a significant number of patients. These antibodies bind to the drug and neutralize some of the drug so that the effective concentration is lower than the total concentration. Some drugs are formulated as a prodrug—an inactive form of the drug that must be metabolized in order to become effective.

There are two routes by which drugs are eliminated from the body: excretion and metabolism. Water-soluble drugs are usually excreted directly through the urine, whereas lipid-soluble drugs must first go through the liver to be metabolized into water-soluble metabolites that may be excreted through the urine. Although drugs may be excreted through the biliary system, intestines, saliva, sweat, breast milk, and lungs, most drug excretion occurs through the kidneys. Renal excretion decreases with age. Bound drugs remain in the blood as only unbound drug can be renally excreted. Un-ionized forms of drugs and their metabolites may filter into the urine, but the kidneys then reabsorb them back into the blood circulation. The biliary tract tends to excrete drugs that are larger, lipid soluble, and conjugated to chemical groups such as glucuronic acid.

7.5 Factors Affecting Pharmacokinetics

Many factors can affect pharmacokinetics. Neonates have a greater proportion of water per kilogram of body weight and higher volumes of distribution for water-soluble drugs. They also have lower drug binding to albumin. Renal clearance is very low at birth and then rises dramatically over the first two weeks before stabilizing. Hepatic metabolism is also low for neonates, because their enzymes are not yet fully functional.

Older patients have a greater proportion of fat per kilogram of body weight and higher volumes of distribution of fat-soluble drugs. They also have lower drug binding to albumin. Renal clearance and hepatic metabolism decrease with age.

Heavier patients usually require higher doses. The relevant type of body weight depends on the medication. Lean body mass may be more appropriate for highly water-soluble drugs that have limited fat distribution and total body weight may be more appropriate for highly lipid-soluble drugs.

Pregnancy can significantly change a number of important physiologic parameters and add a number of potential side effects.

Certain genetic differences such as in cytochrome P_{450} can influence drug absorption, distribution, and elimination. Concomitant medications and certain types of food such as green vegetables or grape juice can also affect metabolism.

7.6 Dose–Response Curves

Most responses are continuous and dose dependent, with the response usually increasing as you increase the dose. Clinical trials generate dose–response data points and a curve is drawn or extrapolated between these points, allowing you to predict responses for doses not tested (e.g., if 4-mg and 5-mg doses were tested, the line between these points would predict the response for a 4.5-mg dose).

However, some responses are not dose dependent and therefore do not conform to a dose–response curve. Classic examples of non-dose-dependent responses are the toxicities such as agranulocytosis and Stevens Johnson syndrome, which can occur at any dose and are neither more likely nor more severe at higher doses.

Some interventions have biphasic (there are two plateaus in the dose response curve) or multiphasic responses. For example, some antibiotics just inhibit the replication of bacteria (bacteriostatic) at low concentrations but actually kill existing bacteria (bactericidal) at higher concentrations. Less commonly, the dose–response curve is U-shaped; that is, as you increase the dose, the effect increases until a peak is reached and then the effect decreases. The low-dose stimulation and high-dose inhibition phenomenon that generates U-shaped curves is called *hormesis*. For example, both very low and very high cholesterol levels are unhealthy. U-shaped curves also result when interventions have agonist (i.e., promotes the effect) activity at certain levels and antagonist (i.e., blocks the effect) activity at other levels.

The standard sigmoidal curve model of efficacy and toxicity is obviously a simplification. Although useful as a starting point, this model has major limitations and relies on some important assumptions. Specifically, the model assumes that:

- Efficacy and toxicity are dose dependent.
- There is not significant variability in response.
- The risk–benefit tradeoff is fixed.
- The dose–response curve remains constant over time.

The first assumption is usually accurate, but there is often a great deal of variability in response from patient to patient, and the risk–benefit tradeoff depends on the type of intervention, disease, and toxicities. You may be less willing to risk a toxic effect if the disease is not life threatening, there are many alternative interventions, or the toxic effect is severe. Conversely, you may be more willing to risk a toxic effect if the disease is life threatening, there is a dearth of alternative treatments, or the toxic effect is mild. For example, in evaluating a blood pressure medication, your tolerance for a severe toxic effect like fulminant liver failure is very low. So the average toxicity curve is not very helpful. Instead, you want to identify the dose at which you are 99.999% sure that fulminant liver failure will not occur. On the other hand, for a medication treating acute myocardial infarction, the acceptable risk of intracranial hemorrhage toxicity may be higher (such as 1%). As to the fourth assumption, we have already discussed the shortcomings.

7.7 Types of Dosing

7.7.1. Flat Doses

A flat dose (i.e., the same dose for all patients) is acceptable for interventions with wide therapeutic windows or for situations with limited heterogeneity. When possible, flat doses are preferable because they are relatively simple and convenient to administer. An example of a flat dose medication is Tylenol. Everyone takes the same dose, despite his or her weight, age, height, ethnicity, or gender. If you cannot seem to identify an acceptable flat dose, sometimes changing the way you measure intervention quantity can help.

7.7.2 Dosing Based on a Baseline Characteristic

Doses can be adjusted on the basis of baseline characteristics. The most common method of adjusting a dose is to use a physiological parameter such as weight (e.g., total weight, lean weight, or estimated weight), body surface area, sex, age, and other physiological parameters. The choice of the physiological parameter depends on the drug and patient characteristics and the efficacy and toxicity parameters (e.g., using total weight rather than lean weight may be better for a drug that distributes largely into fat).

The second most common way of adjusting dose is by metabolism, distribution, or excretion parameters that may affect a drug's therapeutic effects. Adjusting doses for renal or hepatic function (e.g., decreasing doses when either or both are impaired) is relatively common. For highly protein-bound drugs, adjusting doses for serum albumin levels may be important.

A third way of adjusting doses is by disease severity or subtype. More severe forms or different manifestations of a disease may require higher doses. Finally, drug doses may need adjustment in the presence of other drugs because of potential drug–drug interactions.

7.7.3 Titrated Dosing

Titrated dosing involves following a certain parameter and altering the dose to achieve a target value of the parameter. There are three general ways of titrating doses:

- Pharmacokinetics: When simple physiologic parameters such as weight cannot predict a drug's pharmacokinetic activity, you can monitor plasma or serum drug concentrations (e.g., peak, trough, or average) and alter your doses to achieve certain ranges.
- Pharmacodynamics: For example, you can dose heparin to the partial thromboplastin time.
- Clinical effect: Clinical effects or responses can guide dosing (e.g., titrating analgesic doses to pain levels) for both efficacy and safety (e.g., titrating medication doses to liver function test elevations or nausea) if they are immediately apparent, easy to monitor, and reversible (because you can only titrate doses to something that can change).

7.8 Traditional Dose-Escalation and Dose-Ranging Studies

Conventional Phase I studies consist of single ascending dose and multiple ascending dose studies. A single ascending dose study starts with a single low dose administered to a small group of subjects (usually three to six patients). This starting dose should be multiple orders of magnitude lower than the expected efficacious or toxic doses. You can also give placebo to one to two patients. If the data indicate that this starting dose is safe, the dose is increased carefully. The dose continues to be escalated carefully until you either reach maximum safe doses as predicted by pharmacokinetic calculations or start to see unacceptable side effects.

A multiple ascending dose study is similar to a single ascending dose study, except that each patient receives a dose multiple times at some sub-chronic interval over a period of time. The frequency and duration of dosing as well as the length of follow-up after dosing depend on the anticipated dosing schedule in clinical practice, the nature of the disease, anticipated onset of action, and potential for rebound effects, long-term toxicity, and long-term benefit. In a Phase I multiple ascending dose study, giving the drug for four to five half-lives is typical.

In order to protect patient safety, the initial dose in a Phase I study should be very low, typically, 1/25th to 1/100th of the no-effect dose seen in animals. The doses are then escalated.

Typically, dose escalation involves making large dose jumps early on when doses have no effects and making the jumps smaller and smaller as the doses start causing biological effects. For example, if you see no effect at 1 mg, you may jump to 5 mg. If there is still no effect, you could jump to 10 mg. Seeing some effect at 10 mg suggests that the next dose be more cautious.

- Doubling Method: Increase dose by 2× each time.
- Modified Fibonacci Sequence: The first dose is n, the second dose is $2n$, the third dose is $3.3n$, the fourth dose is $5n$, the fifth dose is $7n$, the sixth dose is $12n$, the seventh dose is $16n$, and so forth.
- Log Scale: In this scheme, the dose increases logarithmically: if n is the starting dose, then the next dose level is $10n$, followed by $100n$, then $1000n$, and so forth.
- Half Log Scale: In this scheme, the dose increases half-logarithmically: if n is the starting dose, then the next dose level is $3n$, followed by $10n$, then $30n$, and so forth.
- Accelerated Titration Design I: Each dose level is 40% higher than the preceding dose level.
- Accelerated Titration Design II: Each dose level is 100% higher than the preceding dose level. In either design, each dose level is given to a single (different) patient. When you detect a dose-limiting toxicity, give that dose level to a total of three patients. Then escalate the dose by smaller increments.

To illustrate, the modified Fibonacci sequence where the doses are increased by factors is outlined below in Table 7.1.

TABLE 7.1

Modified Fibonacci Sequence

Doses	Escalation	Example
First dose	First dose	1 mg
Second dose	First dose × 2	2 mg
Third dose	Second dose × 1.67	3.3 mg
Fourth dose	Third dose × 1.5	5 mg
Fifth dose	Fourth dose × 1.4	7 mg
Sixth dose	Fifth dose × 1.33	9.3 mg
Seventh dose	Subsequent dose increased by 1.33	12.4 mg

The modified Fibonacci sequence is, strictly speaking, not a Fibonacci sequence, modified or not, but that is what it is called.

Before testing any doses, you should establish dose-escalation rules: what dosing levels you plan to give and how you will decide whether and when to move to a higher dose level. The disease, potential toxicities, and dose–toxicity curves in animals can help determine your dose-escalation plan. Faster escalation may be appropriate for severe life-threatening diseases with relatively few treatment options. Dose escalation should be much more gradual when there are potentially severe toxicities. In general, you should remember that even during clinical trials you want to avoid giving patients unnecessary, ineffective treatments.

The parallel dose–response design entails randomly assigning patients to one of several groups and giving all patients in each group a specific fixed dose. You may either start the patient on the final or maintenance dose immediately or gradually titrate up to the final dose (in a scheduled forced titration). Demonstrating a positive-sloped dose–response curve suggests that the drug has an effect, even without a comparison placebo group. But you need a placebo group (or some other type of appropriate comparison group) to delineate the actual magnitude of the drug effect. Moreover, when you do not test a wide enough dose range, the dose–response curve might not have a positive slope and only including an adequate control group will reveal that the intervention has an effect.

The crossover dose–response design gives each patient group one dose for a specified duration followed by a different dose for the same duration. Therefore, each patient receives more than one dose level, allowing you to estimate individual and population dose–response curves. This design also requires fewer patients than a parallel group design. However, this design is not ideal for interventions that cause very slow or irreversible responses and for diseases that change over time.

In the forced titration design, you give each patient a stepwise progression of dose escalations. Often, a parallel design placebo group serves as the control group. In the optional titration (placebo-controlled titration to endpoint) design, you also give each patient increasing doses but only until you see a specific favorable or unfavorable response (e.g., a PK, PD, or clinical endpoint). You should always include a concurrent placebo group.

There are four main reasons why the forced dose and optional dose titration designs are most frequently used. First, practicing physicians often titrate doses (e.g., a physician will move the dose of an anti-hypertensive medication up or down depending on the patient's blood pressure). Second, the two titration designs use much fewer patients than the parallel or crossover designs, which is especially important when recruiting patients is difficult (e.g., the disease is rare or the intervention causes toxicity). Third, giving the same patient multiple doses will allow you to plot individual dose–response curves (in addition to population dose–response curves) which is important when interpatient variability is high (i.e., different patients tend to have different responses). Finally, titration studies can identify dose levels for subsequent parallel or crossover studies.

However, the titration designs have several important drawbacks. Time-dependent effects can confound results. Distinguishing among dose–response (i.e., due to dose level), exposure–response (i.e., due to length of time on a treatment), and cumulative dose (i.e., due to total cumulative dose) effects can be very difficult. Diseases that change over time can cause problems as well (e.g., is the better response due to the disease naturally improving or the increased dose?). Moreover, the titration designs do not work well with delayed or very slow responses.

The optional titration design has a particularly important bias. Because patients who do not respond will get higher doses, and because there is usually some variability in response for most diseases the design may spuriously lead to dose escalation raise the target or suggested dose. As a result, higher doses always will have deceivingly high response rates. False-positive responders (i.e., patients who appear to have a response but really do not) will stop dose escalation too early. False-negative nonresponders (i.e., patients who do not appear to respond but really do respond) will continue dose escalation for too long. Therefore, comparing the study group is important and will help identify patients who are less likely to respond to the intervention.

Reference

Chin, R. and Lee, B.Y. 2008. *Principles and Practice of Clinical Trial Medicine*. Elsevier. St. Louis, MO.

8

*Adaptive Dosing**

8.1 Adaptive Dose Finding

One of the advantages of adaptive study designs is that they can yield a much richer set of data than non-adaptive designs. Because of this, they are particularly suited for dose-finding studies, and several techniques have been developed for this purpose. A richer set of data is helpful for dose finding because, unlike efficacy endpoints in a confirmatory or hypothesis testing trial where there is a binary answer as to whether the drug works, there is almost never one right dose. With adaptive trial designs, more data can be collected where they will provide the most value, as can be seen in Figure 8.1.

Also, adaptive dose finding is particularly useful in oncology studies. For oncology studies, patients rather than volunteers are usually enrolled because of the high likelihood of toxicity from the chemotherapeutic drugs. Also, in oncology studies, the drugs are dosed to much higher levels of toxicity than in non-oncology studies. Because the studies are performed in patients who will likely die, and possibly die faster if they are treated with an ineffective drug, and because of the toxicity, it is more important in oncology studies to reach the therapeutic dose faster and minimize the number of patients who are exposed to ineffective doses. Also, it is more likely that overshooting the dose will be fatal or cause grievous injury with chemotherapeutic drugs, so minimizing the overshoot is just as important.

Dose responses almost always have variability from person to person and from one demographic (sex, age, etc.) to another. Dose–response can also be affected by concomitant medications, food, and other covariates and can change over time. Tolerance, or *tachyphylaxis*, can develop.

Also, the therapeutic window may be different for different diseases and patients, as can the risk–benefit the patient is willing to accept. Patient-to-patient variability can be very important and can render the risk–benefit ratio much more acceptable or less acceptable. For example, if the therapeutic window is narrow but the drug has highly predictable bioavailability, it may be much safer than one that has a wide therapeutic window but also a wide variability in absorption.

---

* Parts of this chapter are adapted from Chin and Lee, 2008. With permission.

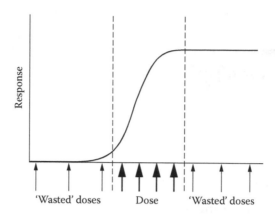

FIGURE 8.1
Adaptive designs can collect more data in more appropriate fashion. (Reprinted with permission from J. Orloff, *Nature Reviews Drug Discovery*, 8:949–957, 2009).

Also, the relationship between dose and exposure is variable, as is the relationship between exposure and effect. Correlating these three moving parts—dose, exposure and effect—can be difficult.

Because of these factors, it is often imperative to not just identify a dose that is safe and effective but also to characterize it in terms of variability, covariates, excretion in renally impaired patients, age, and so on. It is often necessary to identify the minimally effective dose and maximally tolerated dose. All of these goals are often well served by adaptive designs and modeling.

Just as with other parameters, dosing for a drug can be changed on the basis of blinded or unblinded data. And it can be changed during confirmatory trials or during Phase I/II (learning) trials. In most cases, however, adaptive changes in dosing are most helpful in exploratory or "learning" Phase I and II studies. At those phases, unblinded data can be more easily used without statistical concerns.

In fact, adaptive changes in dosing in Phase I studies are standard and in most cases are necessary to achieve the objectives of the study. Adaptive changes in dosing for Phase II studies are not common today but can make a lot of sense and present little statistical difficulties if performed correctly. Changes in dosing during Phase III (confirmatory, adequate, and well-controlled, pivotal) studies can pose the same difficulties of study integrity and interpretability that other adaptive changes based on unblinded data can face.

Some of the earlier adaptive designs were D-optimal designs. These were designs meant to maximize the amount of information about the dose response. These designs maximize the benefit to future patients who stand to benefit from the results of the study but could expose the patients in the study to a higher level of risk because the doses could be aggressively increased. Some of the newer designs, such as continual reassessment method, are more concerned with individual ethics than collective ethics, and properly so. They minimize the risk to the patients in the study and sometimes maximize benefit to those patients. In general, it is inappropriate to expose patients in clinical studies to increased risk of harm if it can be avoided, even at the cost of making the information less helpful for the benefit of the broader patient population.

Successful dose selection and exploration should achieve certain criteria (i.e., performance criteria). It should produce dose–response curves that are detailed (i.e., many data points) and wide (i.e., explores a large range of parameters such as age, renal function, etc.) and define a space with good separation between safety and efficacy (even while accounting for individual variation) while maximizing convenience.

8.2 Phase I Studies

At first glance, you might be tempted to regard all Phase I pharmacokinetic studies as adaptive studies. The standard Phase I studies—single ascending dose, multiple ascending dose studies—appear to be sequential studies (described below). You administer a dose, check for effects, and, depending on the effects, either proceed to a higher dose or stop.

However, such studies primarily compare different dose groups with each other and often do not compare doses versus controls. And the classic designs sometimes do not allow modifications in the dose escalation, sample sizes, or other parameters. They also often do not take into consideration any response or efficacy data.

So rather than sequential studies, many Phase I pharmacokinetic studies are actually nonparallel group design or (if the same patient is dosed repeatedly with different doses of the drug) within-group crossover/modified Latin square design studies. In other words, these Phase I studies are conceptually the same as running a multiple-arm study with a different dose in each arm, except that the arms are conducted sequentially rather than in parallel because of safety concerns. Insofar as these inflexible studies allow for termination of the study for safety reasons, they are adaptive but not very much so.

Modern Phase I studies often are much more sophisticated and take advantage of adaptive design tools to a greater degree. They will often change the dose-escalation scheme in response to the outcome. They will add or subtract patients from dose groups. They will often deescalate as well as escalate. They will often incorporate placebo groups.

Because Phase I studies are exploratory rather than confirmatory, there is no need to preserve alpha. Nor is there, strictly speaking, a requirement to maintain a blind, although in order to reduce the bias of placebo effect, it is advisable to do so.

8.3 3 + 3 and Related Designs

The 3 + 3 design is a common Phase I study design used most often in oncology studies. As previously mentioned, adaptive designs have been in use in oncology studies for a long time. One of the factors that lend oncology studies to 3 + 3 or other adaptive designs is that the unmet need is so great that it is typical to dose anticancer drugs to very high doses that will cause a nontrivial rate of severe adverse reactions. In fact, many oncologists have believed until recently that toxicity and efficacy of chemotherapeutic agents were closely linked.

The standard 3 + 3 design proceeds in the following manner.

- Start with 3 patients at the starting dose.
  - If 0/3 patients have a dose-limiting toxicity, escalate to the next higher dose.
  - If 1/3 patients has a dose-limiting toxicity, treat 3 more patients at the same dose level.
- If 1/6 patients has a dose-limiting toxicity, escalate to the next higher dose level.
  - If >1/6 patients has a dose-limiting toxicity, deescalate to the previous lower dose level.
  - If >1/3 patients has a dose-limiting toxicity, deescalate down to the previous lower dose level.
- If a dose has been deescalated:
  - If only 3 patients have been treated at the dose level, treat 3 more patients.
  - If 6 have already been treated at the dose level, stop the study and declare the dose a maximally tolerated dose.
- The maximally tolerated dose is defined as the highest dose with 1/6 or less dose limiting toxicities observed.
- Escalation never occurs to a dose if that dose has 2 or more dose-limiting toxicities already.
- If 2 or more dose-limiting toxicities occur at the starting dose level, then the study is terminated.

Two versions of the 3 + 3 rule are the traditional escalation rule (TER) and the strict TER (STER) shown in Figures 8.2a and 8.2b. As you can see, TER and STER assume that a greater than 33% incidence of toxicity is unacceptable. Some situations may justify raising (e.g., the intervention is for a severe disease so that higher risk of toxicity is tolerable) or lowering (e.g., the toxicity is so severe or the disease is mild and not life threatening) this threshold.

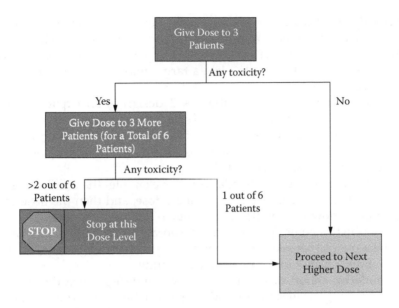

FIGURE 8.2a
Traditional escalation rule (TER). (Reprinted from Chin 2008. With permission.)

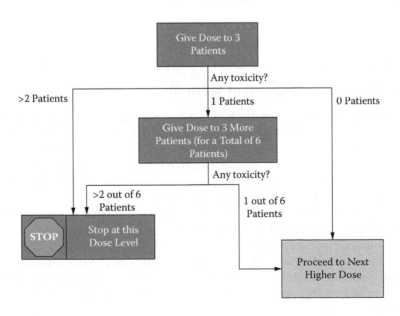

FIGURE 8.2b
Strict traditional escalation rule (STER). (Reprinted from Chin 2008. With permission.)

Obviously, the design does not have to be 3 and 3; it could be 4 + 4 or 10 + 5 or any other permutation. A more general form of the 3 + 3 design is called A + B design or *group up and down designs*. The parameters for escalation and deescalation can be changed to yield a target maximally tolerated dose or other desired doses.

Another possible variation of the 3 + 3 design is an expanded cohort design, where a 3 + 3 design is used to select the maximally tolerated dose and then that dose is further characterized with enrollment of additional patients, with adjustments up or down as necessary. The adjustments can be driven by Bayesian calculations (Ji 2007).

The adjustments can also be adapted. For example, the 3 + 3 design can be used to identify the maximally tolerated dose, and then the dose can be adjusted up or down in smaller increments to fine-tune the dose.

More sophisticated designs would incorporate efficacy parameters as well as the relationship between efficacy and safety. Other designs could use gradations of response or toxicity to guide the study.

A cumulative cohort design is similar to the designs already discussed, in that it preassigns rules for escalation, deescalation, and additional enrollment based on the cutoffs in the dose limiting toxicities. However, unlike the simpler designs, the design incorporates into each decision point not just the current cohort but all patients in the study who have been treated with the dose in question (Ivanova et al. 2007). A cumulative cohort design is nearly as powerful as the continual reassessment model technique discussed below and can be adapted for time-to-event studies.

8.4 Continual Reassessment Method

The continual reassessment method is a Bayesian-based technique for dose finding well suited for Phase I studies that have been widely used and even more widely discussed among statisticians (O'Quigley et al. 1990). It can be considered to be a type of response-adaptive randomization. Its use has been curtailed by a somewhat highly mathematical basis for the technique that is not readily understandable to many clinicians.

Though advocates of the continual reassessment method have argued that the technique puts fewer patients at risk in the higher doses and increases speed, others have expressed concerns that the continual reassessment method may result in very rapid escalation of dosing, to the possible detriment of patients. In fact, the continual reassessment method is a tool that when used correctly can yield benefit to patients but when used incorrectly can be hazardous.

The basis for the continual reassessment method is that the data from each patient are used to predict the dose–response curve for the drug. That dose–response curve is then used select the next dose. In fact, the process largely mimics what happens in clinical practice and many other facets of life, where data from each experience shape what clinicians or others do next. A more descriptive name for continual reassessment method would be *trial-and-error method of exploring doses.*

A continual reassessment method study starts with a tentative dose–response curve that is based on previous animal and other data. In Figure 8.3, that would be the solid curve. A target maximally tolerated dose is selected. For example, you might want a dose that causes dose-limiting toxicity in 25% of the patients. So based on the curve, you dose the first patient with a dose that is expected to have a 25% likelihood of causing dose-limiting toxicity. If you see a dose-limiting toxicity, you would shift the curve upward (larger dotted line), and if you do not, you would shift the curve downward. Based on the new curve, you would dose the patient at the dose you expect to result in a 25% chance of dose-limiting toxicity. After multiple iterations, you should arrive at a dose that is close to the actual dose that causes a 25% rate of dose-limiting toxicity.

Of course, one of the risks of this design is that unlike traditional Phase I studies that introduce a very low dose cautiously at the beginning of the study and gradually escalate, the continual reassessment method could introduce the initial patients to a very harmful or fatal dose. Because of this, a modified continual reassessment method has been introduced, where the

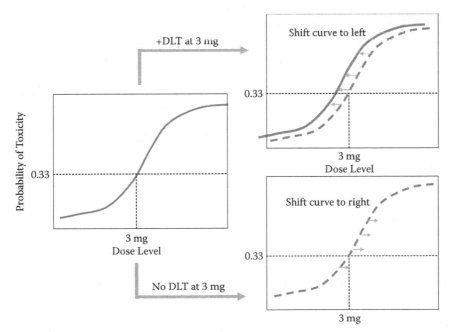

FIGURE 8.3
Continual reassessment method model. (Reprinted from Chin. 2008. With permission.)

study initially begins with a traditional single ascending dose or 3 + 3 design until the first dose-limiting toxicity is seen, after which the design switches to the continual reassessment method.

In addition, rather than changing doses after each patient, some modified continual reassessment method designs treat several patients at each dose. This reduces the likelihood that some patients may be treated with doses that overshoot the target dose by a significant margin.

Furthermore, by putting limits on the size of dose changes at each step, the risk of overdosing can be limited even more.

The traditional continual reassessment method is designed for instances where the dose-limiting toxicity drives the choice of dose and therefore is appropriate for oncology studies. It also normally requires a binary toxicity measure—a measurement that yields either a yes or no. It is not designed for adverse events that are finely gradated, unless a cutoff to make it a binary outcome is used. Also, the shape of the curve is assumed to be continuous, and the toxicity rate is assumed to increase with the increasing dose.

There is a technique called a *time-to-event continual reassessment method* (TITE-CRM), proposed by Cheung and Chappell (2000), which can be utilized for time-to-event studies. In this technique, the patients who have not yet experienced toxicity are entered into the model by giving them credit for the length of time they have been enrolled without a dose-limiting toxicity. That way, they can contribute to the shape of the curve even before they experience an event. This allows enrollment of patients even before the previous cohort has reached their endpoints. A further refinement of this model allows more precise weighting of the patients who have not experience the event by estimating how long it takes for a typical patient to experience an event (Braun 2005).

A continual reassessment method can also be used for efficacy outcome. The limitation of the technique is that it is necessary to decide what the target efficacy rate should be, because the continual reassessment method models the dose that would produce the target effect rate. On the one hand, it could be argued that 100% response is the desired outcome for most diseases, in which case the modeled dose will be very high. On the other hand, you could argue that 100% efficacy is likely to result in unacceptable toxicity. You have to decide what efficacy rate is likely to produce an optimal ratio of benefit and risk. This is not easy.

Of course, this choice of target rate can be a problem in some cases with targeting toxicity as well. In oncology studies, a target toxicity rate of 20% may be the desired dose because with traditional chemotherapeutic agents drugs are dosed to toxicity. Drugs for less severe diseases will not be dosed in the same fashion. A more useful outcome measure may be an optimal relationship between efficacy and safety outcome. For example, the probability of improvement in asthma symptoms minus the probability of a skin rash could be modeled and optimized using the continual reassessment method.

Additional versions of the continual reassessment method can allow dosing based on multiple parameters. For example, if you were performing a cholera challenge study where a volunteer is administered a dose of cholera toxin and a dose of a drug, the continual reassessment method could be adjusted to find the optimal dose for any given dose of the toxin and any given dose of the drug.

Or the continual reassessment method could be designed to optimize dose based on a biomarker or a combination of a biomarker and a clinical outcome. A biomarker is a measurement such as level of a protein or blood pressure that is correlated with clinical outcome. Biomarkers can be a classifier biomarker, prognostic biomarker, or predictive biomarker. A *classifier biomarker* is a baseline marker that is fixed, such as HER2 status. A *prognostic biomarker* predicts the outcome, regardless of treatment. A *predictive biomarker* is a surrogate.

If a drug is intended to produce a clinical outcome that correlates with a biomarker/surrogate, then the biomarker/surrogate can be used to find the dose. If a biomarker is or may be predictive of response, continual reassessment method modeling can take into account both factors and help find a dose that optimizes the outcome for a subgroup with a biomarker response.

As with other dose-finding techniques, the continual reassessment method can be used in crossover studies as well or in studies where a patient receives several different doses.

In the *low, medium, and high* continual reassessment method, instead of administering the same dose to all patients in the same cohort, multiple doses are assigned to them initially. This method will treat fewer patients at low, possibly ineffective, dose levels when the initial levels are far below the true maximally tolerated dose.

8.5 Dose Escalation with Overdose Control

Dose escalation with overdose control is a non-model-based, fully adaptive approach to Phase I studies, most commonly used in oncology studies (Babb 1998). With dose escalation with overdose control, the goal is to limit the number of patients who are likely to be overdosed. You accomplish this by taking information generated from the study and using Bayesian statistics to predict what dose levels will yield what probability of overdosing the patient. You select the dose level so the likelihood of the next patient receiving an overdose is no higher than a set rate, known as the *feasibility bound*. Dose escalation with overdose control is easier to understand and appears to be safer than the continual reassessment method, in that fewer patients will likely be overdosed and experience excess dose-limiting toxicity.

Of course, there are patient-to-patient differences that can affect response and toxicity. A further refinement of dose escalation with overdose control is dose escalation with overdose control with covariates (Wijesinha and Piantadosi 1995). With this technique, information about patients, such as renal clearance, is entered into the model to improve its predictability.

8.6 Stochastic Approximation Methods

Another method that can be used for Phase I dose finding is the stochastic approximation method (Anbar 1984). Stochastic approximation is a statistical technique that was developed to adaptively elucidate the true signal when there is a lot of noise. It is in some ways ideally suited for dose finding because the variability in response from patient to patient (noise) is exactly what the technique is designed to overcome. The algorithms are well worked out, and the technique works as follows: a data point is generated, such as a dose–response; then, based on the response, the dose is changed in the direction that the algorithm predicts; then another dose response is generated; then the dose is changed again but by a smaller amount.

8.7 Summary of Single-Parameter Models

The various techniques to adapt dosing based on responses and toxicities can certainly improve the quality of information from a Phase I trial, protect patient safety, and perhaps improve the likelihood that the patients enrolled in the trial may benefit. However, because Phase I trials are small, the techniques often cannot be fully exploited. The use of these techniques has not been as widespread in Phase II as it might be, but the potential is great.

Some of these techniques are somewhat abstract, so an analogy or two may be helpful. Imagine that you are playing "The Price Is Right." That is a game show in which you have 30 seconds to guess the price of an item. You guess a price and the host responds "higher" or "lower?" depending on whether the actual price is higher or lower than your guess. The traditional 3 + 3 design and similar up-and-down designs would be analogous to guessing in $100 increments up or down. Say the price is $545. You would guess as follows, and the answer would be as follows

- "$100!"—and the host says, "higher"
- "$200!"—"higher"

- "$300!"—"higher"
- "$400!"—"higher"
- "$500!"—"higher"
- "$600!"—"lower"

The stochastic approximation technique would start with big changes in the guesses and narrow in on the price, as follows:

- "$100!"—"higher"
- "$1,000!"—"lower"
- "500!"—"higher"
- "$750!"—"lower"
- "$675!"—"lower"
- "$523!"—"higher"

The continual reassessment method technique would try to make the guess as close as possible and based on the expression on the host's face and crowd response, try to get as close to the price as possible each time.

- "$205!"—"higher" and audience groans
- "$496!"—"higher" and audience claps
- "$572!"—"lower" and audience groans a bit
- "$551!"—"lower" and audience applauds

Statisticians who love adaptive trial designs seem to love modeling, and modeling has shown that the continual reassessment method technique may be the most powerful (O'Quigley 1991).

8.8 Additional Models and Methods

With almost all of the above techniques, but especially the Bayesian-based models for predicting the response curve, it is possible to model both the toxicity and efficacy. This means that after each patient or each group of patients, the model can be updated and, based on the model, the dose with the best combination of efficacy and safety can be tested (Thall 2004).

In special studies, such as combination regimen studies, adaptive designs that model the interaction between efficacy and safety and doses of each drug exist and can be used to select the optimal dose (Dragalin 2008).

Multiple Bayesian techniques exist for dose-ranging studies as well and can be useful, but frequentist methods are usually sufficiently developed and better accepted (Whitehead 2004).

Random walk designs are similar to the up-and-down designs discussed above, but instead of a deterministic up-and-down rule, a "biased coin" is flipped to determine the next dose. The bias is a function of the toxicity or response seen to date. These designs are nonparametric and are simple to implement.

Bayesian D-optimal design techniques maximize the ability of the study to estimate the true dose–response relationship. The patients are allocated to doses that will maximize the amount of information about the dose–response rather than try to reach a certain maximally tolerated dose or other dose. Constraints can be placed so that patients are not unduly exposed to toxic doses.

A penalized D-optimal design is a non-Bayesian technique that also maximizes the amount of information about the dose–response curve. It uses a likelihood function rather than a posterior distribution. Like many other designs, constraints can be placed to safeguard patients.

Pharmacologically guided dose escalation is a technique where for each dose level, the AUC is determined, which in turn determines the next dose escalation.

An adaptive treatment switching technique, also called *rescue* or *early escape*, is a design in which the treatment is discontinued or switched in the middle of a study, usually due to lack of efficacy. This is very common in oncology studies. The failure rate and time to withdrawal can serve as efficacy measures but, unfortunately, many designs use survival instead. Survival of these designs is prone to significant confounding, because after the switch, the patient often receives an alternate effective therapy. The early escape design is more appropriate for a progressive and irreversible disease than for a waxing and waning disease. In a waxing and waning disease, distinguishing between a temporary flare versus true deterioration may be difficult.

8.9 Dose Adaptation in a Pivotal Study

Most of the above techniques were developed for use in Phase I studies where alpha preservation is not critical. For changes in dosing for pivotal or confirmatory studies, the dose adjustments must be made in such a way that it preserves alpha. The traditional group sequential methods, where some of the doses are dropped at the interim analysis, are a clean way of achieving this goal. In a frequentist trial, actually changing the dose rather than dropping a dose is difficult without affecting the integrity of the study, and though techniques could be developed for this, they have not yet. For example, the null hypothesis may be that the relationship between dose and response does not follow a certain curve with a certain variance. In that case, the doses could be changed without sacrificing alpha. This remains an area for further development.

8.10 Changes in Concomitant Medications and Procedures

In addition to changes in the dose of the drug being tested, adaptations in concomitant medications may be made as well. Other procedures that might modify the treatment effect can also be made.

References

Anbar, D. 1984. Stochastic approximation methods and their use in bioassay and Phase I clinical trials. *Communications in Statistics - Theory and Methods*, 13:2451–2467.

Babb, J., Rogatko, A., and Zacks, S. 1998. Cancer Phase I clinical trials: Efficient dose escalation with overdose control. *Statistics in Medicine*, 17:1103–1130.

Braun, T.M. 2005. Generalizing the TITE-CRM to adapt for early- and late-onset toxicities. *Statistics in Medicine*, 25:2071–2083.

Cheung, Y. and Chappell, R. 2000. Sequential designs for Phase I clinical trials with late-onset toxicities. *Biometrics*, 56:1177–1182.

Chin, R. and Lee, B.Y. 2008. *Principles and Practice of Clinical Trial Medicine*. Elsevier. St. Louis, MO.

Dragalin, V., Fedorov, V., and Wu, Y. 2008. Adaptive designs for selecting drug combinations based on efficacy-toxicity response. *Journal of Statistical Planning and Inference*, 138(2):352–373.

Ivanova, A., Flournoy, N., and Chung, Y. 2007. Cumulative cohort design for dose finding. *Journal of Statistical Planning and Inference*, 137:2316–2327.

Ji, Y., Li, Y., and Bekele, N. 2007. Dose-finding in Phase I clinical trials based on toxicity probability intervals. *Clinical Trials*, 4:235–244.

O'Quigley, J. and Chevret, S. 1991. Methods for dose finding studies in cancer clinical trials: A review and results of a Monte Carlo study. *Statistics in Medicine*, 10:1647–1664.

O'Quigley, J.O., Pepe, M., and Fisher, L. 1990. Continual reassessment method: A practical design for Phase I clinical trials in cancer. *Biometrics*, 46:33–48.

Orloff, J. 2009. The future of drug development: Advancing clinical trial design. *Nature Reviews Drug Discovery*, 8:949–957.

Thall, P.F. and Cook, J.D. 2004. Dose-finding based on efficacy-toxicity trade-offs. *Biometrics*, 60:684–693.

Whitehead, J., Zhou, Y., Stevens, J., and Blakey, G. 2004. An evaluation of a Bayesian method of dose escalation based on bivariate binary responses. *Journal of Biopharmaceutical Statistics*, 14:969–983.

Wijesinha, M.C. and Piantadosi, S. 1995. Dose-response models with covariates. *Biometrics*, 51:977–987.

9

Interim Analysis and Adaptive Termination of Study and Study Arms[*]

9.1 Overview

Termination of the study or study arms following an interim analysis, if performed with traditional alpha preservation methods, is well accepted by statisticians and regulatory authorities. These traditional designs share a common trait, namely, that the decisions that are taken after the unblinded analysis are to stop or to continue the study. In this chapter, I will discuss these well-understood and well-accepted designs.

9.2 Data and Safety Monitoring Boards

Data and safety monitoring boards (DSMBs), also called *data monitoring committees* (DMC), are independent committees responsible for performing interim analysis of studies and recommending actions to sponsors. They are typically engaged in blinded studies where access to unblinded data is important to make decisions that will affect the course of the study. For example, they may analyze safety data and recommend that the study stop due to safety concerns.

For adaptive studies, one DMC can be charged with both monitoring the safety as well as for recommending adaptations, or two separate committees can be constituted for each purpose. The membership of the DMC typically includes statisticians, clinicians with expertise in the disease being studied, and clinicians with expertise in the adverse events of particular concern. If a single DMC is used, then the composition of the committee should be expanded from a typical DMC to include statisticians and clinicians familiar with adaptive designs.

---

[*] Parts of this chapter are based on Chin and Lee, 2008. With permission.

All DMC members should sign confidentiality agreements. At the first meeting of the DMC, a DMC charter will normally be finalized, and if a chair has not been designated, a chair is elected. The chair should have previous DMC experience. The DMC charter would specify the need for a quorum, voting rules, and other procedural matters.

It is extremely important to have a written procedure for all communication between the sponsor and the DMC in order to safeguard trial integrity. In some cases, an independent third party whose only function is to be the conduit of information between the sponsor and the DMC is used.

Sometimes the DMCs are structured so that they hold an open session at which the sponsor is present and a closed one without the sponsor. The thought is that this will allow the sponsor to answer any clarifying questions from the DMC. In general, this is not a bad idea—it is a terrible idea. It is very difficult to prevent some nonverbal or accidental compromise of the blinding when the sponsor and the DMC members interact face to face. In general, all communication between the DMC and the sponsor should be in a written form. In some cases, the sponsor is represented in the deliberations of the DMC and participates in the decision-making process. Of course, the representative is firewalled from the rest of the sponsor employees in such cases. This is an even worse transgression than direct communication between the DMC and the sponsor and almost never advisable. In cases where the DMC sessions are not exclusively with voting members of the DMC—for example, outside consultants may participate—the DMC may sometimes hold executive sessions with only DMC members.

There is temptation with adaptive trials, where the designs are very new, and the DMC may not be fully conversant with the technical aspects, to insert the sponsor into the recommendation process. A far better option is to constitute the DMC with personnel familiar with adaptive designs.

All analyses prepared for the DMC should be performed by an independent statistician and/or a programmer. Sometimes this is called an *independent statistical center*. In large companies, this could be sponsor employees who are otherwise uninvolved with the study, but it is much better to utilize an independent third party.

The DMC should keep minutes of the meetings, and though in some cases the minutes of the open session may be distributed to the sponsor, it is generally inadvisable to circulate the minutes. Instead, the chair of the DMC should send a letter with the recommendations from the DMC to the sponsor via the liaison (if there is one) or directly.

DMCs should be provided with rate of recruitment, noncompliance, protocol violations, dropouts, completeness of data, cleanliness of data, subgroup distribution, etc. They should be empowered to ask for additional analysis that may be relevant.

It is important to note that, normally, the DMC itself cannot stop the study. It can only recommend to the sponsor that the sponsor stop the study. This is important because the sponsor does not have to follow the recommendation of the DMC.

In addition, the DMC normally can recommend that the sponsor stop the study only on the basis of the scope it has been given, which is defined in the protocol. For instance, if the protocol allows the DMC to stop the study for safety, it cannot stop it for futility. If the protocol calls for the DMC to recommend the best dose, it cannot generally recommend two doses.

Within the scope they are given, however, the DMC has quite a bit of flexibility. If it is charged with stopping the study for safety, and the main concern is about agranulocytosis, for example, it can stop the study for thrombocytopenia if the risk is great enough. The purpose of using a DMC with clinicians, is that it can apply clinical judgment to interpret the data and there would be no point in having a DMC committee if the rules were completely rigid.

9.3 Stopping Rules

With a traditional interim analysis, the trial can generally be stopped for superiority, inferiority, futility, or safety. The techniques for these are well worked out, and there is not much statistical or regulatory controversy about these types of interim analysis as long as they are performed correctly. With more sophisticated designs, arms can be dropped for any of the above reasons without stopping the study, and these are relatively uncontroversial as well (Brannath 2003; Hommel 2001; Kropf 2000; Wang 2001).

As discussed in more detail in Section 3.7, most stopping rules are based on the concept of a boundary. If the results become extreme enough that they cross a statistical boundary, the trial is stopped. The boundaries specify how extreme the results need to be before they need to be stopped. The stopping rules can be based on efficacy, including superiority, equivalence, or noninferiority; or on safety. Although the stopping rules can be based on Bayesian methodology, most are still based on frequentist methods, which have been well accepted by regulators.

9.4 Individual Sequential Designs

In individual sequential designs, also called *fully sequential designs*, results are examined after each patient and the trial is stopped or changed on the basis of the available data. These are used typically for Phase I studies. The principles involved are the same as for the techniques explained below.

9.5 Group Sequential Designs

In a group sequential design study, you administer the intervention or control to a group of patients, analyze the results, and then based on the analysis modify the study for the next patient or group of patients.

Group sequential designs are well understood. They unequivocally preserve alpha and are readily accepted by regulatory authorities.

Historically, the decisions in group sequential designs were go/no-go decisions or drop-an-arm decisions. The studies would be started with two or more arms, an interim analysis would be performed, and if the results indicated that efficacy was overwhelming, safety was unacceptable, or the study was futile, the DMC would recommend discontinuation of the study or an arm. The sponsor would then normally terminate the study or the arm. Though the studies were adaptable in concept and fulfilled the modern criteria for adaptive designs, they were in spirit similar to conventional studies. The decision rules were firmly proscribed and the process for gathering the data, cleaning it, and presenting it was laborious. Sometimes the studies would even need to be placed on hold while the data was analyzed and processed for the interim analysis.

In Section 3.7, the various statistical methods for prespecifying the boundaries for the decision were discussed in detail. The following discussion relies on the statistical techniques reviewed in that section.

The "drop the loser" design involves performing an interim analysis during the course of the study and dropping one or more of the arms that are showing negative or undesirable results. The "play the winner" design is the opposite of the drop the loser design. Instead of eliminating arms that show no or undesirable effects, the play the winner design entails enrolling additional patients into arms that appear the most promising.

The Simon two-stage design is a commonly used oncology study design, typically used for Phase IIa studies. The design relies on enrolling a small number of patients for the first stage, and following them for a specified length of time (while further enrollment in the study is suspended). Based on the number of responses (shrinkage of the tumor) from the first stage, the study is stopped or continues to the second stage. The boundaries for stopping and continuing are based on two alternate hypotheses, one for the top and one for the bottom limits of the response. For example, hypotheses may be "drug has less than 10% response rate" and "drug has more than 40% response rate." Simon two-stage design is relatively efficient, fairly simple to execute, and can be quite flexible.

References

Brannath, W., Bauer, P., Maurer, W., and Posch, M. 2003. Sequential tests for non-inferiority and superiority. *Biometrics*, 59:106–114.

Chin, R. and Lee, B.Y. 2008. *Principles and Practice of Clinical Trial Medicine*. Elsevier. St. Louis, MO.

Hommel, G. and Kropf, S. 2001. Clinical trials with an adaptive choice of hypotheses. *Drug Information Journal*, 35:1423–1429.

Kropf, S., Hommel, G., Schmidt, U., Brickwedel, J., and Jepsen, M.S. 2000. Multiple comparison of treatments with stable multivariate tests in a two-stage adaptive design, including a test for non-inferiority. *Biometrical Journal*, 42:951–965.

Wang, S.J., Hung, H.M.J., Tsong, Y., and Cui, L. 2001. Group sequential test strategies for superiority and non-inferiority hypotheses in active controlled clinical trials. *Statistics in Medicine*, 20:1903–1912.

10

Adaptive Changes in Study Design and Decision Rules

10.1 Overview

As mentioned before, using Bauer's technique of combining p values, derived from meta-analysis, it is theoretically possible to change almost any part of a study design (Bauer 1994). These changes are called *decision rules*. Bauer's and related techniques are controversial and are not well accepted by regulatory authorities. Some of these techniques are outlined in this chapter.

10.2 Changes to Follow-Up Period

Typically, the follow-up period (after the last dose of the drug) in a study is determined in advance. However, sometimes it is not clear how long the effect of the drug will last. In other cases, safety events that occur during the study may necessitate long duration of follow-up. Pharmacokinetics and pharmacodynamics of the intervention may have been poorly estimated at the beginning of the study and the follow-up period may need to be changed.

Adaptive designs can allow for a longer follow-up period based on these and other parameters. Typically, the follow-up is for the purposes of collecting long-term safety data or less commonly to assess return of the disease over the long term. Unless the efficacy is being used to drive the length of follow-up, little statistical risk is incurred with this type of change in study design, because Type I error is unaffected.

10.3 Flexible Designs

With flexible designs, in some cases the study can be terminated at the interim, but other designs such as self-designing approaches do not permit termination of the study at the interim analysis. With flexible designs, changing doses, selecting sites, redesigning multiple endpoints, changing the hypothesis, changing the test statistics, and selecting goals between noninferiority and superiority are all possibilities.

Shen and Fisher (1999) have outlined the variance spending approach for changing the sample size and other features of the trial on the fly without prespecification. Other authors have proposed methods that can also add flexibility based on interim analysis, including Bauer (1994), Lan (1997), Cui (1999), Lehmacher (1999), Chi (1999), Denne (2000), Muller (2001), and Wang (2001).

10.4 Changing the Endpoints and Hypothesis

10.4.1 Changes Based on Blinded Data

The primary endpoint can be modified before the blind is broken if it becomes apparent that the original endpoint is inappropriate. For example, perhaps the primary endpoint was to be a 6-week change in visual acuity but too many patients missed the 6-week visit. The endpoint can be changed to the 10-week change in visual acuity. Or perhaps a separate study demonstrates that there is a strong placebo effect within the first 8 weeks.

Other changes that can be made to the endpoint include definition or composition of the endpoint and changes in the hierarchy of the endpoint testing.

As with other adaptations, the modifications ideally should be rule based and prespecified. For example, the protocol might prespecify that the 6-week visual acuity will be the primary endpoint unless more than 20% of patients miss the visit, in which case 10-week visual acuity will be used. Changes to the protocol based on unexpected data without prespecification in the original protocol do not represent true adaptive clinical trial design but would more properly be termed *reactive clinical trial design*.

Changing the analysis population can be done fairly easily before the unblinding. For example, the primary hypothesis can be changed to apply only to a particular subgroup. This is different from changing the inclusion criteria—this is analyzing only a subset of the patients without necessarily changing patient enrollment.

10.4.2 Changes Based on Unblinded Data

In addition, with flexible designs designed using the Bauer method, the null hypothesis can be changed (Bauer 1994). Switching between noninferiority and superiority designs can be performed with caution, particularly if the switch is from noninferiority to superiority. You can also change the hierarchy of the hypothesis (Hommel 2001).

Under the Bauer rubric, endpoints can be changed during the course of an adaptive study (Bauer 1994). For example, the number of primary endpoints can be changed, endpoints can be dropped or changed, and various other changes can be made. The potential changes include switching or altering primary endpoint weighting.

10.5 Changes to Test Statistic or Analysis

10.5.1 Changes Based on Blinded Data

As mentioned earlier, statistical analysis relies on a set of assumptions. For example, in order to utilize a t test or other parametric tests, the distribution of data must be parametric, or bell shaped. Other assumptions such as similar variance across the groups and linearity of the outcome measure were discussed in Chapter 3. If at the end of the study (or during the study) it becomes apparent that the statistical assumptions are incorrect, then the statistical analysis plan (SAP) may be modified so that the more appropriate statistical analysis can be performed. However, this type of modification is only permissible in a nonadaptive trial if the study blind has been scrupulously maintained, because otherwise, there is great risk that the analysis is being modified in order to change a negative study into a positive one.

Other types of changes that can be made include changes in the plan for transformation of the data (e.g., to make it more linear) and addition of covariates. Similarly, the definition of the per patient population can be changed, and the analysis can be changed from intent to treat to modified intent to treat, for example. If these changes are made before unblinding, there is usually not an issue with statistical integrity.

10.5.2 Changes Based on Unblinded Data

With the Bauer method the test statistic and analysis can be changed based on the interim analysis (Bauer 1994). For example, the shape of the dose–response curve for a dose–response trial can be modified based on the interim data (Lang et al. 2000). Survival studies can be modified from a continuous proportional hazard ratio to one that changes over time or one that has some alternate shape (Lawrence 2002). This can be helpful because many drugs do exert a differential effect in a population over time. For example, cancer vaccines sometimes cause worsening of survival initially and then improve survival. Using an analysis based on a survival curve that reflects such changes in survival would increase the power of the study.

Another adaptation that is possible is to add a covariate to the final analysis if it appears at the interim that the covariate is important in affecting outcome and there might be an imbalance in that covariate (Wang 2005).

Another adaptation that is not usual but would be of great benefit in many studies is adaptation of the location scale test. Most statistical analysis is based on an important assumption that the standard deviation and variance are equal between the arms of the study. With many drugs, the drug will change both the response (location) and the standard deviation (scale). For example, Herceptin increases survival in HER2 overexpressers but not in non-overexpressers. As with other drugs that only work in responders, Herceptin will increase the variance in the treated arm if non-HER2 overexpressers are enrolled.

Now, most Phase III studies that are based on reliable Phase II results should take location scale into account, but this is not always done. For Phase II studies themselves, as well as some Phase III studies, the location scale will not be well studied at the beginning of the study. The location scale assumptions can be adapted at the interim analysis based on the data collected (Neuhäuser 2001).

Also, in cases of reverse multiplicity, where you have multiple coprimary endpoints in a trial, the correlation of the primary endpoint may be different from the original assumptions. In such a case, the analytic methods can be updated. Also, covariates that were not collected sufficiently or for other reason are not useable can be dropped, and the analysis parameters such as the role of various covariates and biomarkers can be adapted on the basis of interim analysis.

Obviously, if trend analysis is being used, adaptive score in the trend analysis can be implemented, and if repeated measures analysis is being used, adaptive change in the model for repeated measures can be implemented.

References

Bauer, P. and Kohne, K. 1994. Evaluation of experiments with adaptive interim analyses. *Biometrics*, 50:1029–1041. (correction *Biometrics*, 52:380, 1996.)

Chi, G.Y.H. and Liu, Q. 1999. The attractiveness of the concept of a prospectively designed two-stage clinical trial. *Journal of Biopharmaceutical Statistics*, 9:537–547.

Cui, L., Hung, H.M.J., and Wang, S.-J. 1999. Modification of sample size in group sequential clinical trials. *Biometrics*, 55:853–857.

Denne, J.S. 2000. Estimation following extension of a study on the basis of conditional power. *Journal of Biopharmaceutical Statistics*, 10:131–144.

Hommel, G. 2001. Adaptive modifications of hypotheses after an interim analysis. *Biometrical Journal*, 43:581–589.

Lan, K.K.G. and Trost, D.C. 1997. Estimation of parameters and sample size reestimation. *Proceedings of Biopharmaceutical Section*, 48–51.

Lang, T., Auterith, A., and Bauer, P. 2000. Trend tests with adaptive scoring. *Biometrical Journal*, 42:1007–1020.

Lawrence, J. 2002. Design of clinical trials using an adaptive test statistics. *Pharmaceutical Statistics*, 1:97–106.

Lehmacher, W. and Wassmer, G. 1999. Adaptive sample size calculation in group sequential trials. *Biometrics*, 55:1286–1290.

Muller, H.-H. and Schafer, H. 2001. Adaptive group sequential designs for clinical trials: Combining the advantages of adaptive and of classical group sequential procedures. *Biometrics*, 57:886–891.

Neuhäuser, M. 2001. An adaptive location-scale test. *Biometrical Journal*, 43:809–819.

Shen, Y. and Fisher, L. 1999. Statistical inference for self-designing designing clinical trials with a one-sided hypothesis. *Biometrics*, 55:190–197.

Wang, S.-J., Hung, H.M.J., Tsong, Y., and Cui, L. 2001. Group sequential test strategies for superiority and non-inferiority hypotheses in active controlled clinical trials. *Statistics in Medicine*, 20:1903–1912.

Wang, S.J. and Hung, H.M.J. 2005. Adaptive covariate adjustment in clinical trials. *Journal of Biopharmaceutical Statistics*, 15:605–612.

11

Seamless Designs and Adaptive Clinical Trial Conduct

11.1 Seamless Designs

With traditional studies, there is usually a gap of 6 to 9 months between the end of one study (defined as last patient out or the collection of the last data point of the study) and the beginning of the next (defined as first patient in or the randomization of the first patient in the study). This time is required to collect the data, clean the data, lock the database, run the statistical analysis, interpret the data, run additional analysis, perform sensitivity analysis, conduct business analysis, design the next study, write the protocol, design the case report forms, label the drug, file the regulatory documents, obtain institutional review board approval, and enroll the patients.

This gap is a significant factor in the length of clinical development process for drugs. With new technology, the gap can be reduced or eliminated. Seamless clinical trials are trials in which there is little or no gap between the end of one study and the beginning of the next.

There are two general categories of seamless designs. *Operationally seamless design* refers to elimination of the gap between two trials even though each trial is a nonadaptive, traditional clinical trial. For example, a traditional Phase II trial might end one week, and a traditional Phase III trial might start the next.

Inferentially seamless design refers to designs where the purpose of two phases of clinical development might be melded into one adaptive design. This often means that the two stages of the trial will be analyzed as one joint study.

Seamless designs require several operational improvements over traditional designs. First, the data collection and processing must be performed rapidly. This is best accomplished with electronic data capture (EDC). Modern EDC systems can make data available within hours of data entry. The EDC system must be coupled with processes that take advantage of its capabilities. It is of little benefit if, for example, the data are available but there are no statisticians to perform the analysis on the data set or if the processes are such that the data analysis takes a long time. The statistical programs must be written and validated in advance, so that as soon as data are available the analysis can be performed. The data cleaning process must be optimized so that the cleaning does not fall behind data entry. The data quality plan must be written with rapid turnaround in mind and not call for unreasonable and generally unnecessary 100% data accuracy.

Second, the trial setup processes must be coordinated and performed in advance so that there is not an administrative delay. If institutional review board/ethics committee approvals need to be performed, regulatory approval must be obtained, or contracts negotiated with sites, then there will be a gap between the trials. The best way to avoid such delays is to write the protocol for the study as one integrated protocol so that the approvals need to be obtained only once. In cases where this is not possible, the protocol can be submitted to the approval bodies in advance with several alternate doses and designs, leaving the exact design variable. Some of the current approval bodies are not yet familiar with adaptive designs, so this process might not be straightforward, but as adaptive designs and seamless studies become more common, the approval process will likely become smoother. Also, it may be helpful to use central institutional review boards that can process the protocol rapidly.

11.2 Challenges in Adaptive Trials

Adaptive clinical trials present particular challenges. First, although integrity of the blinding is important in any study, it is particularly important in adaptive clinical trials because the risk for unblinding is much greater. Second, adaptive clinical trials, especially seamless trials, require rapid collection, processing, cleaning, and analysis of the data. Third, in many cases, the changes after the interim analysis has been completed must often be put into place very rapidly.

11.3 Maintaining the Blind

Of course, it is important to maintain the blind in all clinical studies except for open label studies, but protecting the blind is particularly important and critical in adaptive designs because the risk is much higher than in a traditional study. In addition, it is important to document that the blind has been maintained, to give regulators confidence that the study integrity has been preserved.

The first step in maintaining the blind is to prepare detailed written standard operating procedures (SOPs) that specify who will be exposed to the unblinded data and how the blind will be maintained. They should specify how the unblinded data will be controlled, who will perform the interim analysis, how that interim analysis will be communicated to the DMC, and what the contingencies are in case there is contamination. There should also be clear procedures for how and what information is sent from the DMC back to the sponsor. As with all SOPs, there should be prespecification of how the training of the SOPs will be performed and how compliance will be checked and monitored.

All documentation, including snapshots of the database used for the interim analysis, interim analysis itself, DMC minutes, and similar material should be preserved.

If a clinical research organization is used, the sponsor must make sure that they are qualified and trained properly, and auditing to make sure that they are rigorously following the advisable procedures.

In some cases, inference about the efficacy and safety might be made on the basis of some decision taken at the interim analysis. For example, if the highest dose is stopped, then some people may infer that the highest dose was too toxic. There is no need, if the operations of the study are well designed, for people outside the DM committee to know which dose has been discontinued. There can be transfer of instructions from the DM committee through the sponsor to the drug supply vendor or personnel that a specific arm needs to the discontinued without disclosing which dose it is.

Nevertheless, it is unavoidable that in some cases, inference of efficacy and safety may be impossible to prevent.

11.4 Infrastructure and Operations

There are several critical factors for success of adaptive trials. The first is planning. Because adaptive trials can diverge in multiple potential directions in terms of size, dosing, and protocol changes, it is critical for the team to plan carefully for contingencies and to have enough available buffer. The buffer applies to both materials, such as drug supply, as well as to personnel. You should keep in mind that some of the personnel whose availability may be required on short notice include people outside the direct team, such as the contracting group who may need to process amendments to the site contracts on short notice or institutional review boards that might need to process protocol amendments on short notice. The team must always be thinking several months ahead.

The second is an experienced team. The team members must have experience in clinical trials and ideally in adaptive clinical trials. The optimal team is a dedicated team that works only on that study, but nondedicated team members shared with other projects can work as long as their time is carefully budgeted and they can respond in real time to project needs. It is also very important to have a statistician who understands adaptive designs and can perform simulations for both clinical data and for resource and logistics planning. The simulations should test different recruitment speeds and clinical outcomes.

For forecasting resources, including personnel, it is helpful to use critical chain project management (CCPM) rather than simple project management. CCPM takes into account not just tasks that need to be completed and their dependencies but also the resource sharing across and within projects. Simple project management often fails to consider the competing demands on the time of project team members and will render inaccurate forecasts because of this. CCPM can be performed using many of the standard project management software.

Excellent information technology is also very helpful for adaptive designs. State-of-the-art clinical drug supply systems, modern interactive voice response system (IVRS) that can be adapted and validated quickly, data management systems that can process data rapidly, and clinical trial management systems that can handle adaptive designs are all important. Ideally, the software such as IVRS should be self-validating as much as possible so that changes to the study are not subject to often lengthy debugging and validation processes.

Data analysis programs should be self-validating as much as possible as well, so that new analysis can be done on the fly without laborious manual validation. Data analysis programs should also generate sensitivity analysis automatically because interim analysis will often be based on data sets that are incomplete or not fully cleaned. Excellent data management will minimize the amount of uncleaned or incomplete data, but there is no requirement that the data be completely clean before each interim analysis.

Managing drug supply can be a particular challenge, especially with dose-ranging studies that might call for changes in dose strengths midway through the study. It is helpful to have an automated drug labeling and packaging system with automated validation so that changes can be made as necessary. In many cases, four or five dose strengths, if selected with foresight and spaced appropriately, can cover a wide range of doses. Alternatively, multiple dose forms can be prepared in advance and shipped as required, but the cost can be prohibitive in such cases.

Adaptive studies can be very challenging for clinical sites. Instructions can change repeatedly, and they may have difficulty keeping up with the changes. Frequent retraining, in person or via the Web, is helpful in making sure that the sites stay up to date. Monitoring visits should focus on changes to the protocol and procedures and ensure that the sites, pharmacies, and laboratories are up to date with the latest changes in the study. It is often helpful to have a checklist generated for each patient from the Web interface so that the site coordinators can rely on up-to-date personalized instructions.

Adaptive allocation of monitoring effort is becoming more common even with nonadaptive studies, but given the importance of risk management and directed monitoring for adaptive designs, adaptive monitoring and data cleaning is highly recommended.

Because the length and size of the adaptive study is sometimes not fully specified at the beginning of the study, it is important to specify the payment schedule to the investigators and to the clinical research organization in a manner that can accommodate changes in the protocol. The contracts can specify the payment schedule based on one of several potential scenarios or based on work units. A contract specialist is always helpful for such contracts but is particularly important for adaptive trials where the workload is not fixed. In fairness, clinical research organizations and sites should receive some compensation if the study is terminated early, because they will have allocated part of their capacity to the study.

11.5 Adaptive Trial Protocols

The U.S. Food and Drug Administration (FDA) has issued some specific guidelines regarding adaptive design protocols and submissions (FDA 2010). In order to evaluate an adaptive design protocol, they require that the sponsor provide not just the protocol but also study procedure documents, including DM committee or other committee charters. They also require material used by the sponsor to justify and plan the study. These include simulations performed to design the study and background material such as statistical papers used for the design of the study. Of course, the SOPs for maintaining the blind are required.

The FDA is in general not in favor of completely flexible designs. They strongly prefer that each of the potential interim analyses be planned in advance and a full description of the potential adaptations, the criteria for the adaptations, and the statistical treatment of the adaptations be prespecified. They also require "the assumptions made in the study design with regard to these adaptations, the statistical analytical approaches to be used and/or evaluated, the clinical outcomes and quantitative decision models for assessing the outcomes, the relevant calculations that describe treatment effects, and the quantitative justifications for the conclusions reached in planning the trial."

They require a full SAP in advance, including planned endpoints, design, criteria for success, hypotheses, testing procedures, data management, and quality plan (FDA 2010). The documentation submitted to the FDA should include discussion of the following which is excerpted from the 2010 FDA Guidance:

- A summary of the relevant information about the drug product, including what is known at the present stage of development about the drug from other studies, and why an adaptive study design, in contrast to a nonadaptive design, has been chosen in this situation. The role of the chosen adaptive study design in the overall development strategy should also be discussed.

- A complete description of all of the objectives and design features of the adaptive design, including each of the possible adaptations envisioned, assumptions made in the study design with regard to these adaptations, statistical analytical approaches to be used and/or evaluated, clinical outcomes and quantitative decision models for assessing the outcomes, relevant calculations that describe treatment effects, and quantitative justifications for the conclusions reached in planning the trial.

- A summary of each adaptation and its impact upon critical statistical issues such as hypotheses tested, Type I errors, power for each of the hypotheses, parameter estimates and confidence intervals, and sample size. In general, the study design should be planned in a frequentist framework to control the overall study Type I error rate. A Bayesian framework that incorporates uncertainty into planning parameters in a quantitative manner (i.e., prior distributions on parameters) can also be useful for planning purposes to evaluate model assumptions and decision criteria. If models are used to characterize the event rates, disease progression, multiplicity of outcomes, or patient withdrawal rates, these models should be summarized clearly to allow evaluation of their underlying assumptions. Summary tables and figures should be included that incorporate all the important quantitative characteristics and metrics that inform about the adaptive design.

- Computer simulations intended to characterize and quantify the level of statistical uncertainty in each adaptation and its impact on the Type I error, study power (conditional, unconditional), or bias (in hypothesis testing and estimates of the treatment effect). The simulations should consider the impact of changes in a single design feature (e.g., the number of dose groups to be dropped), as well as the combination of all of the proposed adaptive features.

    The computer programs used in the simulations should be included in the documentation, as should graphical flowcharts depicting the different adaptive pathways that might occur, the probabilities of their occurrence, and the various choices for combining information from the choices. For example, the following quantitative models can be used to reflect various study features considered in evaluating the stages of an adaptive design and the impact of combining information from each of the stages:

- Models for study endpoints or outcomes.
- Models for the withdrawal or dropout of subjects (e.g., for lack of compliance, toxicity, or lack of benefit).
- Models of the procedure for selecting among multiple study endpoints (e.g., selection of the types of events included in a composite endpoint).

For each design evaluated with simulations, the documentation should clearly describe the following:

- A listing of all branching options possible at each stage of adaptation along with the chances of selection of each option.
- Various design features and assumptions.
- Event rate background.
- Entrance criteria and event rate association with such criteria.
- Subgroup differences or heterogeneity in response.
- Procedure for combining data on treatment effects from different stages of the study, including any weightings.
- Statistical methods for estimation of treatment effects at each study stage and at final study completion along with the statistical bias in the estimate.
- Statistical calculations of the Type I error properties of the design at each study stage and at final study completion and the calculations of study power.
- Full details of the analytic derivations, if appropriate. For some adaptations, statistical calculations of the Type I error and/or statistical bias in treatment effect estimates can be performed analytically without using simulations. If the analytic approaches are based on published literature, the portions of the analytic approaches specifically relevant to the adaptive design employed should be provided in detail.

The composition, written charter, and operating procedures for the personnel assigned responsibility for carrying out the interim analyses, adaptation selection, and any other forms of study monitoring. This information should include all of the written agreements that the sponsor has in place and written assurances from the involved parties for the protection of information that should not be shared outside of the limited team with access to the unblinded data. A description of whether a sponsor-involved statistician will perform the unblinded analysis and/or whether sponsor-involved personnel (e.g., sponsor employees or contract research organization (clinical research organization) staff) will make recommendations for the adaptation should be included. A well-trusted firewall established for trial conduct beyond those established for conventional group sequential clinical trials can help provide assurance that statistical and operational biases have not been introduced.

For submission of study reports, the FDA requires a study conduct report, including a description of deviations from the adaptive plan, snapshots of the databases used for the adaptations, copies of the analysis, a copy of the final database, analytic methods, sensitivity analysis, tests for consistency across the stages of the study, as well as standard statistical analysis required for conventional studies.

Reference

Food and Drug Administration. 2010. *Guidance for Industry: Adaptive Design in Clinical Trials for Drugs and Biologics.*

12

Analysis and Interpretation of Results*

12.1 General Issues in Interpretation of Clinical Trial Results

There are some key principles that are important in interpretation of any study. They apply to the interpretation of adaptive designs. These are summarized in this section.

Interpretation of a trial consists of two steps. The first step is assessing internal validity of the study. This is the process of figuring out what the results tell us about the drug's effectiveness within the trial. The second is external validation or the process of taking the study results and extrapolating them to the patient population at large, to patients who were not entered in the trial. It is the process of reaching conclusions about how the therapy should or should not be used for patients in clinical practice.

To put it another way, if the study shows that the intervention had an effect on the primary endpoint, among the sample of patients in the study, it has internal validity. If the study design, conduct, and results are such that the results can be extrapolated to the population from which the sample has been drawn, the study is said to have external validity.

In addition, there are often ancillary questions that are part of data interpretation. These include questions such as, "If the study was negative, why was it negative?" and "What do the data tell us about the next study to conduct?"

The processes of study interpretations and external extrapolation are highly dependent on the quality of execution. Faulty study design, sloppy execution, and erroneous data analysis can all have a highly detrimental effect. Therefore, part of data interpretation is to recognize and flag those flaws and to determine what impact they have on the interpretations and conclusions, as well as to determine whether there are ways to correct or ameliorate the flaws. Some of these can make an enormous difference in the interpretation of the study.

One of them is protocol adherence. You want to make sure, for example, that the patients had the disease of the type and severity that the study was designed for. You want to make sure that the diagnosis was correct and that the appropriate tests and imaging were done as per protocol, so that you can assure

---

* Part of this chapter is based on Chin and Lee, 2008. With permission.

yourself and others that the appropriate patients were enrolled. Enrolling the appropriate patients is not a straightforward proposition. In many studies, many investigators enroll patients who are not eligible or who do not have documentation that they have the disease. Making sure that the patients meet the inclusion and exclusion criteria is a critical part of study interpretation.

You also want to make sure that the patients received the drug and received the drug at the right does at the right times. You also should check that the assessments of drug effect, especially the primary endpoint assessments, were conducted at the right times. You should also check that the appropriate validation and calibrations were performed on the instruments and that the study personnel were trained and certified appropriately. In short, you should verify that the patients were the appropriate patients; that they were treated and assessed properly; and that there is appropriate documentation to that effect.

Finally, you should verify that the appropriate laws and regulations were followed. For example, it is extremely important to verify that informed consents were obtained properly, because it would be unethical to use the data otherwise.

As a general rule, it is good practice to "pressure test" the results of the study for robustness. Certainly, regulatory agencies such as the U.S. Food and Drug Administration (FDA) will typically perform these pressure tests. These tests fall into two categories. The first examines the data to detect anomalies that might suggest underlying problems with the design, conduct, or interpretation of the study. The second changes assumptions used in the analysis to generate sensitivity analysis of the data.

For example, one of the most important assessments is to examine missing data and missing patients and to determine whether there is a pattern in the missing data; whether the quantity of the missing data is so large that it threatens the validity of the study; whether the results change if different imputation methods are used; and so on. Another typical assessment is to examine thoroughly the baseline demographics to determine whether there are baseline imbalances. There will always be some imbalances, but it is rare that they are significant enough to affect results. What you will be looking for are signs that randomization was performed incorrectly or in a biased fashion.

Subgroup analysis is also often performed, to determine whether there are certain groups of patients to whom the study results may not be applicable or whether there might be a problem with the study. The subgroups typically include those of a certain sex, age, geography, or from a particular site but may also include patients who were enrolled in the first half of the study vs. in the second half or with one manufacturing lot of the drug vs. another and so on.

If the endpoints in the study are not well established and well validated, they must be validated in the study. One of the first steps in interpretation of the results should be examination of the validation data to ensure that the measures are reliable, reproducible, and valid.

A common mistake comes from selecting an inappropriate endpoint. One mistake that is more subtle but devastating is selecting an endpoint that is subject to competing risk, sometimes called *survivor bias*. For example, if one were examining the rate of congestive heart failure after a myocardial infarction, the patients who received tenecteplase (tPA) would have a higher rate than patients who received a placebo. This is because patients who would have otherwise died without tPA survived after receiving tPA but survive with compromised ejection fraction. In other words, the number of patients with congestive heart failure increases because the number of patients who die decreases and instead become congestive heart failure patients.

Sometimes there are artifacts that negate the study results. For example, you might find that the treatment effect emerged during the screening period, before any intervention was administered. As another example, in cancer studies using progression-free survival, the timing of the study visits and computed tomography (CT) scans has a very important impact on time to event. Progression, or growth of the tumor, is generally detected at the time of the CT scan. If the randomization and schedule visits are such that patients in the placebo arm happen to have an earlier visit schedule (even by a few days) in one arm, those patients will tend to have faster apparent progressions even if the active drug has no effect on survival.

Finally, you should make sure that placebo was truly inactive. In some cases, placebo or a supposedly inactive component of the placebo formulation may have a beneficial deleterious effect on the study endpoints. For example, if you are testing cyclosporin for cystic fibrosis and you have propylene glycol in your placebo solution, this may introduce an artifact because propylene glycol may exacerbate cystic fibrosis.

As mentioned previously, statistical tests are based on assumptions. These include assumptions of linearity, assumptions of minimal sample size, and so on. Unless the statistician is alerted when the assumptions are violated, he may not make appropriate adjustments to the methods. An example would be using a parametric test when the samples are not parametric. Another would be to use a standard test such as a *t* test when there are only a few patients in the sample. Another would be to assume equal variance when the variances are not equal. Another would be to treat noncontinuous measurements such as EDSS as if they were continuous measures.

Another example would be to ignore biological nonlinearity, such as with blood pressure, and use tests that rely on linearity assumptions. Blood pressure has a U-shaped curve with relation to cardiovascular outcome in myocardial infarction patients. Very low pressure is a poor prognostic indicator, as is very high blood pressure. Unless a statistician is alerted to this fact, he is liable to apply methods designed only for linear relationships to the blood pressure data, with resultant misleading conclusions. As another example, hazard function is usually assumed to be constant over time, but this is not always the case. For example, for cardiovascular bypass surgeries, the mortality rate is the highest right after surgery and then rises again a few days after surgery.

Another would be to ignore biological collinear relationships. Many biological processes are interlinked, and collinearity is a very common phenomenon. Most statistical tests, however, assume an absence of collinearity. For example, it would be inappropriate to perform an analysis of atrial fibrillation paroxysm frequency without correcting for number of episodes that occur in the same patients, because one paroxysmal episode often increases the likelihood of a repeat episode. If you assume that each episode is independent, you are likely to end up with an inaccurately low p value, because a handful of patients having multiple episodes might skew the data.

Another very common mistake is to utilize inappropriate imputation. For example, if multiple patients drop out of a study because they are feeling so good as a result of receiving the drug that they are no longer motivated to continue in the study, imputing all missing patients as failures would lead to misleading results. Imputation may be required for patients who, though they did not drop out, must be excluded from analysis because they did not meet the inclusion/exclusion criteria, did not receive the drug, received a prohibited drug, or for other reasons.

Subgroup analysis is useful for understanding limitations of the drug but not for extracting evidence of efficacy in a negative study. It should not be used for primary analysis unless prespecified. Any time you analyze a patient population that is different from the one that was randomized, you can introduce a bias.

Completer analysis includes in the analysis only patients who completed the study. *Responder analysis* includes only patients who responded to the drug. *Pharmacodynamic responder analysis* is the practice of including only patients who had a biological response to the drug in the analysis. One example would be to include only patients who raised antibodies against a vaccine in the analysis. *Pharmacokinetic responder analysis* is similar, except only patients who had adequate levels of drug absorbed are included in the analysis.

Per protocol analysis includes only patients who did not have protocol violations or who did not have major protocol violations in the analysis. Except for per protocol analysis, which can occasionally be valid, the other analyses listed here can be very misleading.

A p value in and of itself tells you whether there was a significant effect on the outcome but does not tell you how large the magnitude of the outcome was. In clinical practice, you want to know not just whether the drug impacts outcome but also how much difference it makes. A drug that reduces cholesterol by 1% is very different from one that reduces it by 50%.

For this reason, point estimates and confidence intervals are often used to describe the effect of the intervention on the primary (and other) endpoints. Point estimate is the best guess regarding how much effect the treatment has or what the value of the parameter being estimated is. The confidence interval describes how confident you are about the point estimate; a 95%

confidence is typically used, and it is a measure that describes the values in-between which you would expect the true value to lie in 95% of the cases.

Point estimate plus confidence interval is often preferred over a p value because the point estimate is an indication of how much effect there is, and the confidence interval is an indication of how strong (statistically) the likelihood of difference is. The first is driven by the effect of the drug and the second is driven by the size of the study. This is in contrast to the p value, which collapses the two (how well the drug works and how large the study is) into one value.

The objective of a clinical trial is to deliver results that can be used to improve patient care. In the final step of interpretation, the conclusions from the study are extrapolated to the patient population at large and beyond the narrow hypothesis being tested. In this step, external validity is asserted.

However, most studies are conducted on a sample of patients. In every case, the sample differs from the overall patient population in some respect, either intentionally or inadvertently. The study procedures and patient care should be as similar to clinical practice as possible, but these too can never be identical to clinical care. Endpoints used in the study should capture as much of the disease burden and impact as possible but they, by necessity, must be a distillation of the full spectrum of disease burden.

Therefore, at the end of a study, you must examine the results along with the study design and study conduct and determine how the results can be applied to the patient population at large. This is a tall order. The conclusions must be based on reliable and high-quality data. The analysis must be free from fallacies or technical mistakes. The results must be convincing and robust to sensitivity analysis, and the confidence intervals must be acceptable. The results must be relevant to clinical endpoints. The endpoint must be broad enough to encompass or represent the main aspects of a disease. The risk–benefit ratio must be acceptable. The patient population, the way in which the study was conducted, and the way in which the patients received care must be similar enough to the patient population at large so that the results will be generalizable.

This dichotomy between the trial results and real life is sometimes described as *efficacy vs. effectiveness*. Efficacy is whether a drug in a rather artificial situation of a clinical trial, particularly a blinded randomized clinical trial, shows clinical effect. Effectiveness is whether it has a clinically meaningful effect in the practice setting.

The first step in assessing external validity is to compare the patients in the study, both intended and actually enrolled, against the intended patient population. The goal of a trial is to enroll a broad range of patients, with the hypothesis that the patients are homogeneous and that they will have a homogeneous response. Results of a study are only directly applicable for the group of patients with the same severity and type of disease, time course, concomitant medications, stage of disease, and dosing. They may be indirectly applicable to patients who are not exactly analogous.

You should ask:

- Do the inclusion criteria reflect the target population?
- Do the exclusion criteria bias the results, making them inapplicable to certain portions of the population?
- Were all clinically important clinical criteria considered?

The primary endpoint of a trial is often expressed in a dichotomous fashion: positive or negative. Either the trial met its endpoint or it did not. However, the ultimate utility of a trial depends on a host of factors, including the risk–benefit ratio. Did the magnitude of the benefit outweigh the magnitude of the side effects? More broadly, did the magnitude of the benefit outweigh the cost, inconvenience, known side effects, and the potential unknown (as of yet) side effects?

In order to make this determination, several factors come into play.

First, you should determine much benefit was observed. This is *not* the same as a p value. It is possible to achieve very small p values with a trivial clinical benefit if the sample size is large enough. For example, an increase in walk distance of 10 m may have a p value of 0.01 with a sample size of 100, and the same increase might have a p value of 0.00001 with a sample size of 5,000.

Second, was the benefit seen in everyone, or was there a subgroup that benefited the most? Is it possible to predict who will benefit? Does the benefit accumulate over time? Is there tachyphylaxis? Is there rebound?

In other words, you should determine how much benefit there is and how it is distributed among the patients. You should also determine whether there are ways to maximize the magnitude of the benefit.

Next, you should examine the safety profile. What were the adverse events that were observed? Is it possible to determine who is at risk of the harm? Is it possible to detect the adverse event early and perhaps early enough to treat it?

Just as with efficacy, you should determine how many safety issues there are and how they are distributed among the patients. You should also determine whether there are ways to minimize the impact of the adverse events.

However, one aspect of safety makes the risk–benefit assessment asymmetrical. Though efficacy is often fairly well defined from the clinical study, risk is almost always incompletely defined. This is because most studies are not large enough to characterize the safety profile well. Just as no drug is 100% safe, no clinical study or program will completely characterize the safety profile. Therefore, when assessing the risk–benefit, you must be cognizant that you are weighing the known benefits against both known and as-yet unknown risks.

As you are drawing the final conclusions, you should keep in mind some of the classical mistakes that many people make in drawing conclusions from a study. Some of the mistakes arise from the inherent design of the study.

For example, confirmation bias is the tendency to look for confirmatory evidence and not for evidence to disprove one's assumptions, and it tends to be common—cognitively, humans tend look for data to confirm their prior beliefs and ignore the ones that tend to refute it. This is often true in clinical trials. For example, it may be noted that a headache seems to develop in patients who have had coffee with the drug. One of the first things that a researcher would do would be to determine whether stopping the coffee would decrease the incidence of headaches. What they do not do is stop the sugar or start patients on coffee—an experiment that if positive would refute the hypothesis.

Some of the mistakes arise from rescue bias, which is the tendency to find faults in the study to invalidate it if the results are not as expected; example would include finding that the patient population selected is not representative or that the blinding was inadequate.

Auxiliary hypothesis bias is similar to rescue bias but, rather than invalidating the results of the study, this is the tendency to try to limit the generalizability of the study—that had the wrong dose been used, or the follow-up been longer, the patients been younger, etc. the study results would have been different. Mechanism bias is a similar bias and is related to what happens with multiple comparisons and refers to the natural human tendency to accept even a spurious result if it makes sense.

12.2 Interpretation of Adaptive Trial Results

In addition to the caveats that apply to clinical trial results in general, there are some caveats that apply to adaptive trials. First, many adaptive designs call for early termination of the study or study arms. With early terminations, there is a bias toward overestimation of the results. Because extreme results are more likely to result in early termination, and because results/ estimate of the effect will vary in the course of a study, the likelihood is that if a study is terminated because the results cross a statistical boundary, the point estimate based on that result will likely be more extreme than the true value. This is true for both efficacy- and safety-driven terminations.

This illustrates one of the issues with adaptive designs. Many of the adaptive designs are excellent for disproving or failing to disprove a hypothesis, but the actual estimate of the effect of the drug can be challenging or misleading in some cases. As mentioned before, if significant aspects of the study are adapted, such as the primary endpoint or inclusion criteria, it can be very difficult to estimate the treatment effect or even to understand what the clinical conclusion from the study should be.

Another potential pitfall is modeling. Modeling is often used in adaptive designs, such as a continual reassessment method. Modeling can be very attractive in making sense of data that may be otherwise unintelligible, but limitations of modeling must be understood and recognized. Modeling is a simplification of the data, for one, and, as with other simplifications, may result in the loss of some of the richness of data. In addition, modeling is usually highly dependent on assumptions that go into the construction of the model. For example, in modeling dose–response curves, assumptions about the shape of the curve must be made—whether it is a linear response, sigmoidal, etc. These assumptions have an enormous impact on the results of the modeling. And these assumptions are not easy to get right. For certain stereotyped modeling such as dose–response, self-modeling techniques that may remove some of the subjectivity from the modeling process have potential, but these statistical techniques have not been fully developed yet.

In adaptive designs, covariate adjustments are often also made. Covariate adjustments are also highly prone to the assumptions and the techniques used. You have to decide which covariates have an impact on outcome and which do not. You also have to decide how and in what order the covariate adjustments will be made. Changing the order of the adjustments can sometimes result in different results. If some of the covariates are correlated with each other (i.e., they are not independent), you can end up overadjusting for the covariates.

Both modeling and covariate adjustments can introduce a bias into the results that are dependent on the person(s) performing the analysis. They introduce an element of subjectivity that can bias the study and affect study integrity. To some extent, this risk can be mitigated by prespecifying some of the techniques in advance before the data become available, but the risk cannot be completely eliminated.

As with covariate adjustments, restricted randomization can also introduce a bias, in that sometimes it can increase rather than decrease imbalances. Stratified and adaptive randomization can in theory cause underinflation of effect and also bias if there are unknown covariates that are correlated with one of the stratified covariates.

12.3 Documentation of Trial Integrity

It is unfortunately not uncommon that blinding is broken either inadvertently or on purpose in the course of the study. IVRS errors are unfortunately not rare either, and this can be devastating to the study. Labeling errors and misdosing errors are also seen in many studies. Instrument errors or errors in labeling and shipping of laboratory samples are also seen in many studies. All of these affect trial integrity. In a complicated adaptive design, it is particularly important to protect the integrity of the study and to document that the integrity has been preserved.

12.4 Statistics of Adaptive Trial Analysis

Apart from trial integrity, prevention of Type I error is the greatest area of scrutiny for adaptive studies. A great deal of development in the field of statistics has resulted in a number of effective tools for preventing inflation of Type I error. However, many of the tools are new and unfamiliar to many statisticians and nonstatisticians. Some of the tools are controversial and somewhat immature. It is very important that the statistical techniques are well understood before, during, and after the study so that they can be properly applied.

In addition to alpha control techniques, some tools for analysis of adaptive trials are novel or atypical as well; for example, use of exact tests or randomization tests. When trials undergo adaptation, there is greater possibility that the distribution of data will not be normal. For example, a change in the inclusion criteria may result in two subgroups that are somewhat different, and the distribution of data may be bimodal. One option in such cases is to use nonparametric tests that are valid for nonnormal data distribution. These tests are less powerful than parametric tests.

Another option is to use exact tests (also called *randomization tests* or *permutation tests*). Exact tests rely on calculating the *p* value by examining every possible permutation of outcome. For example, if there are 20 patients per arm in two arms, and each patient could have two outcomes, the exact tests would examine every possible permutation of patients and outcomes. Exact tests become too complicated to compute for large sample sizes.

For large sample sizes, however, a Monte Carlo simulation or other simulation can render a reasonably accurate distribution of data that resembles the actual potential distribution. With such techniques, analysis can be performed for nonnormal distributions that are more powerful than generic nonparametric tests.

With dose-finding studies, extensive use of modeling can provide the best, though imperfect, way to analyze the data.

One of the issues in adaptive trials is that the adaptations can cause changes in patient populations or responses. In fact, the purpose of adaptations is often exactly to accomplish those outcomes. In analysis of the results, however, the differences between pre- and postadaptation should be characterized, because the differences can be illustrative of how the drug works and can help with application of the results to clinical practice. However, interpretation of adaptive studies often will be more difficult than traditional studies. For example, with flexible designs, the null hypothesis can be changed. If the study is positive, the final conclusion is that the first hypothesis is not true in the first group of patients and the second is not true in the second group. It can be difficult to extrapolate that kind of result into the clinical setting.

12.5 Summary

Adaptive clinical trials hold the promise of faster, better, more efficient, and more ethical clinical development. It is a young field and undergoing rapid development. There are still issues that need to be solved, including issues with execution and interpretation of results. However, it is a branch of clinical trial medicine that represents the next major advance in epistemology of medicine and will provide a great service to clinical trialists and patients alike.

Reference

Chin, R. and Lee, B.Y. 2008. *Principles and Practice of Clinical Trial Medicine*. Elsevier: St. Louis, MO.

Index

A

A + B design, 134
Adaptive randomization and allocation,
    101–109
    adaptation of inclusion and exclusion
        criteria based on blinded data,
        107–108
    allocation codes, 103
    balancing (covariate) adaptive
        randomization, 104–105
    Bayesian randomization, 107
    bias, introduced, 101, 103
    combination and multimodal
        randomization, 106–107
    disease progression, 109
    distribution of covariates, 104
    "drop the loser design," 106
    fixed or static allocation, 101
    group demographics, 101
    inclusion criteria, change in, 107
    patient enrichment adaptations,
        108–109
    placebo, 104
    "play the winner design," 105
    randomization, 101
    response (outcome) adaptive
        randomization, 105–106
    restricted and blocked
        randomization, 102–103
    run-in periods, 108
    simple randomization, 102
    stratified, nested, and similar
        randomization, 103–104
    subgroups dropped, 108
    traditional fixed allocation, 101–102
Adequate and well-controlled (A&WC)
    studies, 75
Allocation, *see* Adaptive randomization
    and allocation
Alpha
    preassigning, 39
    preservation, 27, 143
    spending function, 64

Analysis and interpretation of results,
    163–173
    auxiliary hypothesis bias, 169
    clinical trial, objective of, 167
    completer analysis, 166
    compliance with regulations, 164
    computed tomography scans, 165
    confidence intervals, 166
    covariate adjustments, 170
    documentation of trial integrity, 170
    efficacy vs. effectiveness, 167
    equal variance, assumption of, 165
    exact tests, 171
    faulty study design, 163
    inclusion criteria, change in, 171
    instrument errors, 170
    interpretation of adaptive trial
        results, 169–170
    interpretation of clinical trial results,
        163–169
    Monte Carlo simulation, 171
    permutation tests, 171
    pharmacodynamic responder
        analysis, 166
    pharmacokinetic responder analysis,
        166
    placebo, 165
    point estimates, 166
    pressure test, 164
    randomization tests, 171
    rescue bias, 169
    responder analysis, 166
    statistics of adaptive trial analysis, 171
    stereotyped modeling, 170
    subgroup analysis, 164
    summary, 172
    survivor bias, 165
    tachyphylaxis, 168
    tenecteplase, 165
    unethical use of data, 164
Auxiliary hypothesis bias, 169
A&WC, studies, *see* Adequate and well-
    controlled studies

B

Background, 1–36
  adaptations, types of, 10
  adaptive design example, 9
  alpha preservation, 27
  analogy, 9
  antineoplastic agents, 2
  asthma drug, 9
  automated cell counters, 14
  binary answers, 16, 19
  case report forms, 4
  classification and terminology of
      adaptive clinical studies, 20–21
  clinical trials, phases, 2
  communication systems, 14
  comparator drug, 8
  computer processing power, 13
  confirmatory studies, 18
  confirming trials, 16, 17
  confirm type of trials, 13
  costs, escalation of, 1
  covariate analysis, 11
  customized printing, 14
  cytochrome P450 gene, 7
  data entry edit checks, 13
  data and safety monitoring boards,
      11
  definition of adaptive clinical trial,
      5–10
  definition and history of traditional
      clinical trials, 2–5
  descriptive trials, 16
  differential bias, 23, 24
  dose titration, 12
  Down Syndrome patients, 7
  drug efficacy, 19
  drug safety, 15
  drug toxicity, 3
  electronic data capture, 13
  enzyme replacement therapy, 12
  ethics, 15
  evolving regulatory environment for
      adaptive clinical trials, 27–30
  exposure–response analysis, 19
  flexible clinical trial, 6
  fully sequential designs, 20
  inclusion criteria, narrow, 26
  individual sequential designs, 20

interactive voice response systems, 14
internal validity, 23
investigational new drug application,
    34
iterative analysis, 13
last observation carried forward
    analysis, 12
learn and confirm, 12, 16–20
learning phase trials, 16
learning study, 18
limitations of adaptive clinical trials,
    21–22
liquid chromatography–mass spec
    techniques, 14
logistics considerations, 26
lupus patients, 25
modeling, 19
new enabling technologies and other
    requirements for adaptive
    trials, 13–14
non-adaptive study, 8, 21
nuisance parameters, 27
null hypothesis, false, 23
patient safety, 25
performance criteria for well
    designed clinical trials, 22–27
pharmacodynamics, 2
pharmacokinetics, 2
phase evolution, 3
precursors to modern adaptive
    clinical trials, 10–13
Provenge Phase III study, 21
rationale for adaptive clinical trials,
    14–15
regulatory authorities, 22
regulatory guidance from FDA,
    30–36
  early and middle period of drug
    development, 31
  evaluating and reporting
    completed study, 34–36
  late stages of drug development,
    31–32
  special protocol assessments, 32–33
  study blinding and information
    sharing, 33–34
seamless designs, 15
self-designing studies, 9
simulations, 5

special protocol assessments, 28, 31, 32
standard operating procedures, 33
statistical methods, 5
study, validity of, 1
study databases, 35
study-wide error, 23
systematic bias, 23, 24
tables, listings, and graphs, 13
therapeutic–response curve, 17, 18
uninterpretable result, 23
Web-based tools, 1
Bayesian statistics, 30, 40
Bell-shaped curve, 53
Bias
  auxiliary hypothesis, 169
  biased coin, 140
  differential, 23, 24
  introduced, 101, 103
  rescue, 169
  statistical, 90
  survivor, 165
  systematic, 23, 24
Biomarker(s)
  antibody as, 99
  classifier, 137
  definition of, 137
  design modification based on, 78
  predictive, 137
  prognostic, 137
Bonferroni correction, 60, 61
Bootstrapping, 73
Boundaries approach, 64

C

Carryover effect (drug), 120
Case report forms (CRFs), 4
CCPM, *see* Critical chain project management
Cell counters, automated, 14
Central limit theorem, 52
CI, *see* Confidence interval
Classifier biomarker, 137
Clinical trials, *see* Trial
Communication systems, 14
Comparative statistics, 43
Completer analysis, 166
Computed tomography (CT) scans, 165

Computer processing power, 13
Conditional error function, 65
Conditional power, 115
Confidence interval (CI), 69
Confirming trial, 16, 17
Covariate analysis, 11
CRFs, *see* Case report forms
Critical chain project management (CCPM), 158
CT scans, *see* Computed tomography scans

D

Data entry edit checks, 13
Data monitoring committees (DMC), 143
  accruing study data, 74
  member confidentiality agreements, 144
  sponsor, 144
Data safety monitoring board (DSMB), 11, 62, 98, 143
Decision rules, 149, *see also* Study design and decision rules, adaptive changes in
Decision trees, 73
Descriptive statistics, 41
Deterministic models, 72
Differential bias, 23, 24
Distribution model, 73
DMC, *see* Data monitoring committees
D-optimal design, 130, 140
  Bayesian, 140
  penalized, 140
Dose
  escalation, 125, 126
  groups, dropping of, 77
  individualization of, 119
  –response curves, 17, 18, 122
  selection studies, 81
Dosing (adaptive), 129–141
  3 + 3 and related designs, 132–134
  A + B design, 134
  abstract techniques, 138
  adaptive dose finding, 129–131
  adaptive treatment switching technique, 140
  additional models and methods, 139–140

biased coin, 140
biomarker, definition of, 137
changes in concomitant medications
    and procedures, 141
classifier biomarker, 137
continual reassessment method,
    134–137
cumulative cohort design, 134
D-optimal designs, 130
dose adaptation in pivotal study,
    140–141
dose escalation with overdose
    control, 137–138
early escape, 140
efficacy outcome, continual
    reassessment method used for,
    136
ethics, individual vs. collective, 131
feasibility bound, 137
group up and down designs, 134
non-Bayesian technique, 140
oncology studies, 136, 140
Phase I studies, 131
predictive biomarker, 137
prognostic biomarker, 137
rescue, 140
single-parameter models, 138–139
stochastic approximation methods,
    138
tachyphylaxis, 129
tolerance, 129
traditional escalation rule, 132, 133
Dosing (traditional), 117–127
    antibody formation, 121
    biological effects, 125
    carryover effect, 120
    cholesterol levels, 123
    comorbid conditions, 118
    crossover dose–response design, 126
    definitions and objectives of dose
        selection, 118–119
    dose escalation, 125, 126
    dose–response curves, 122–123
    factors affecting pharmacokinetics,
        122
    fat-soluble drugs, 122
    forced titration design, 126
    frequency of dosing, 120
    hormesis, 123
        issues, 119–120
        margin of safety, 119
        modified Fibonacci sequence, 126
        older patients, 122
        patient safety, 117, 125
        pharmacokinetics, 120–121
        placebo group, 127
        protein-bound drugs, 124
        risk–benefit ratio optimization, 119
        risk quantification, 119
        Stevens Johnson syndrome, 122
        therapeutic ratio, 119
        titration studies, 127
        toxic effect, life threatening disease
            and, 123
        toxicity, prediction of, 118
        traditional dose-escalation and dose-
            ranging studies, 124–127
        types, 123–124
            dosing based on baseline
                characteristic, 124
            flat doses, 123
            titrated dosing, 124
        water-soluble drugs, 121
"Drop the loser" design, 106, 146
Drug(s)
    carryover effect, 120
    comparator, 8
    cumulative effect, 120
    delayed effect, 120
    difficulty in evaluating, 95
    efficacy, 19
    fat-soluble, 122
    FDA approval, replication
        requirement, 28
    overnight delivery of, 13
    protein-bound, 124
    safety, 15
    supply, management of, 158
    toxicity, 3
    water-soluble, 121
DSMB, *see* Data safety monitoring
    board

E

EDC, *see* Electronic data capture
EDSS score, *see* Expanded disability
    status scale score

Efficacy vs. effectiveness, 167
Electronic data capture (EDC), 13, 155
EMA, *see* European Medicines Agency
Error(s)
    instrument, 170
    spending approach (sample size
        reestimation), 113
    study-wide, 23
    Type I, 23
        avoided, 23
        control, 6, 20, 76
        frequentist rubric, 24
        inflation, 55, 89, 171
        interim analysis and, 6
        preserved, 66
        probability of, 56
        rate, 84
        risk, 22, 61
        statistical calculations of, 161
    Type II, 23
        avoided, 23
        rate, inflation of, 89
        reduced levels, 24
        treatment effect and, 90
        underpowered studies and, 111
Ethics, 15, 25, 131
European Medicines Agency (EMA), 2
Exact tests, 171
Expanded disability status scale (EDSS)
        score, 112

F

Fat-soluble drugs, 121
FDA, *see* U.S. Food and Drug
        Administration
Feasibility bound, 137
Fixed allocation, 101, *see also* Adaptive
        randomization and allocation
Flat doses, 123
Flexible clinical trial design, 66
Frequentist method (statistics), 38–39
Fully sequential designs, 145
Futility, 78

G

Gaussian distribution, 53
Group sequential design(s)
    implementation of, 79
    random highs in, 90
    unblinded interim analyses, 74
Group up and down designs, 134

H

Holm *t* test, 61
Hormesis, 123
Hypothesis
    changing of, 150–151
    -confirming trials, 27
    null, 44–45
        exclusion criteria and, 70
        frequentist method, 38
        statement of, 45
    Phase III testing of, 3
    rejected, 47
    testing, 6, 44

I

IND, *see* Investigational new drug
        application
Independent statistical center, 144
Individual sequential designs, 145
Inferentially seamless design, 155
Inferential statistics, 41–43
Institutional review boards, 99, 156
Instrument errors, 170
Interactive voice response systems
        (IVRSs), 14, 158
Interim analysis and adaptive
        termination of study and study
        arms, 143–147
    agranulocytosis, 145
    alpha preservation, 143
    confidentiality agreements, 144
    data monitoring committees, 143
        description of, 143
        member confidentiality
        agreements, 144
        sponsor, 144
    data and safety monitoring boards,
        143–145
    "drop the loser" design, 146
    fully sequential designs, 145
    group sequential designs, 146
    independent statistical center, 144

individual sequential designs, 145
overview, 143
"play the winner" design, 146
statistical boundary, 145
stopping rules, 145
Internal pilot study, 114
Internal validity, 23
Interventional studies, 44
Investigational new drug application
    (IND), 34
IVRSs, *see* Interactive voice response
    systems

L

Last observation carried forward
    (LOCF) analysis, 12
Learn and confirm paradigm, 12, 16
Learning phase trials, 16
Likelihood method (statistics), 40
Liquid chromatography–mass spec
    techniques, 14
LOCF analysis, *see* Last observation
    carried forward analysis

M

Margin of safety, 119
Model(s)
    continual reassessment method, 135
    deterministic, 72
    distribution, 73
    efficacy, 139
    seamless designs, 161
    single-parameter, 138
    toxicity, 139
Modified Fibonacci sequence, 126
Monte Carlo simulation, 72, 171

N

Noninferiority studies, 88
Normal distribution, 53
Nuisance parameters, 27, 112
Null hypothesis, 44–45
    exclusion criteria and, 70
    false, 23
    frequentist method, 38
    statement of, 45

O

Observational studies, 44
Oncology studies, 132, 136, 140
Operationally seamless design, 155
Outcome dependent randomization, 83

P

Parametric tests, 51
Patient
    characteristics, 1, 25
    dropouts, 23
    enrichment adaptations, 108–109
    older, 122
    population
        changes in, 171
        characteristics, 74
        choice, 32
    recruitment, 54
    safety, 25, 117, 125
PD, *see* Pharmacodynamics
Permutation tests, 171
Pharmacodynamic responder analysis,
    166
Pharmacodynamics (PD), 2, 120
Pharmacokinetic responder analysis, 166
Pharmacokinetics (PK), 2, 120, 122
Phase I studies
    alpha preservation, 140
    classic designs, 131
    continual reassessment method, 134
    data collection, 4
    dose escalation, 124, 137
    dosing, 11
    individual sequential designs, 145
    learning trials, 130
    multiple ascending dose study, 125
    oncology studies, 132
    purpose, 2
    risk of, 3, 10, 117
    stochastic approximation method,
        138
Phase II studies
    adaptive changes in dosing for, 130
    designed as hypothesis testing
        studies, 3
    heterogeneity of, 2
    location scale, 152

Phase III studies
    hypothesis testing, 3
    Provenge, 21
Phase IV studies, 2
PK, *see* Pharmacokinetics
Placebo, 46, 104, 165
"Play the winner" design, 105, 146
Posterior distribution, 71
Predictive biomarker, 137
Prior distribution, 71
Prognostic biomarker, 137
Prospective study, 44
Provenge Phase III study, 21

R

Random highs (group sequential
    designs), 90
Randomization
    definition of, 101
    tests, 171
Reactive clinical trial design, 150
Repeated significance tests, 63
Requirements for adaptive trials, *see*
        Specific requirements for
        adaptive trials
Rescue bias, 169
Responder analysis, 166
Restricted sampling rule, 115
Results, interpretation of, *see* Analysis
        and interpretation of results
Retrospective study, 44
Risk–benefit ratio optimization, 119

S

Sample size reestimation, 111–115
    additional rules, 115
    adjustment in follow-up time, 114
    background, 111–112
    blinded data, 112–113
    conditional power, 115
    error spending approach, 111, 113
    expanded disability status scale
        score, 112
    false-negative results, 111
    information-based design, 115
    internal pilot studies, 114
    nuisance parameter, 112

restricted sampling rule, 115
sample size, factors determining, 111
self-designing method, 113
sequentially planned decision
        procedure, 111
statistical power, 114
Type II error, 111
unblinded data, 113–114
underpowered studies, 111
variance-spending method, 113
SAP, *see* Statistical analysis plan
Seamless designs and adaptive clinical
        trial conduct, 155–162
    adaptive trial protocols, 159–162
        computer simulations, 160
        description of objectives, 160
        models, 161
        summary of adaptation, 160
        summary of relevant information,
            160
    challenges in adaptive trials, 156
    critical chain project management,
        158
    documentation, 157
    drug supply, management of, 158
    electronic data capture, 155
    firewall, 161
    inferentially seamless design, 155
    infrastructure and operations,
        157–159
    interactive voice response systems,
        158
    maintaining the blind, 156–157
    operationally seamless design, 155
    payment schedule, 159
    personnel, 157
    regulatory approval, 156
    seamless designs, 155–156
    team members, 157
    trial setup processes, 156
    uncertainty, 160
Self-designing studies, 9, 68
SNK test, *see* Student-Newman-Keuls
        test
SOPs, *see* Standard operating
        procedures
SPA, *see* Special protocol assessments
Special protocol assessments (SPA), 28,
        31, 32

Specific requirements for adaptive
        trials, 95–100
    analgesic administration example, 96
    biomarkers, antibody as, 99
    data safety monitoring board, 98
    difficulty in evaluating drugs, 95
    dropout rates, 97
    endpoint availability, 95
    endpoints in adaptive studies, 95–97
    example, 96
    institutional review boards, 99
    partial data, 96
    placebo-controlled study, 98
    practical requirements, 99
    study length, 96
    surrogate endpoints, 97, 98, 100
    surrogates and biomarkers, 97–99
Standard operating procedures (SOPs),
        33, 157
Static allocation, 101, *see also* Adaptive
        randomization and allocation
Statistical analysis plan (SAP), 62, 151
Statistical bias, 90
Statistics, 37–54
    analogy, 39, 45
    assumptions, 50–54
        background, 50–52
        constant hazard ratio
            assumptions, 53
        continuity and linearity
            assumptions, 53
        independence of events, 54
        independent and random
            sampling, 53–54
        parametric assumption, 52–53
    basic statistics, 37
    Bayesian method, 40
    bell-shaped curve, 53
    biological phenomena, 53
    biological world, variability in, 43
    central limit theorem, 52
    comparative statistics, 43
    confidence intervals, reliance on, 38
    continuous variables, 49
    descriptive statistics, 41
    determinism, 42
    dice sums, 49
    example of inference and hypothesis
        testing, 45–47

    examples of statistical tests, 48–50
    frequentist method, 38–39
    Gaussian distribution, 53
    hypothesis testing, 44
    inferential statistics, 41–43
    interventional studies, 44
    likelihood, 38, 40
    normal distribution, 53
    null hypothesis and standard of
        proof in clinical trials, 44–45
    observational studies, 44
    other schools, 41
    parametric tests, 51
    placebo groups, 46
    population, 41
    preassigning alpha, 39
    precedent event, 42
    prospective study, 44
    rejected hypothesis, 47
    retrospective study, 44
    sample, 41
    statistical schools, 37
    statistical tests and choice of
        statistical test, 47–48
    study termination, 39
    test variable, 47
    traditional clinical studies, 37
    z-test, 50
Statistics, adaptive clinical trials, 55–93
    adaptive clinical trial design, 66
    adaptive methods, 65–69
    adequate and well-controlled
        studies, 75
    alpha description, 56–58
    alpha preservation, 55–56
    alpha spending function, 64
    alpha splitting, 59
    asthma drug, 58
    Bauer method, 66
    Bayesian approach, 71
    Bonferroni method, 61
    bootstrapping, 73
    boundaries approach, 64
    composite event endpoint, 80
    conditional error function, 65
    confidence interval, 69
    confidential information, 79
    COPD patients, 57
    data monitoring committee, 74

data safety monitoring board, 62
decision trees, 73
deterministic models, 72
differential weighting, 85
distribution model, 73
dose groups, dropping of, 77
dose selection studies, 81
endpoint adaptation, 87
evolution of adaptive analytic
    methods (interim analysis),
    62–65
FDA stance on adaptive techniques,
    73–93
    adaptive study designs whose
      properties are less well
      understood, 81–88
    statistical considerations for less
      well-understood adaptive
      design methods, 89–93
    valid approaches to
      implementation, 74–81
Fisher-based method, 66
flexible approach, controversy of, 67
flexible clinical trial design, 66
futility, 78
Holm t test, 61
ICU hospitalization, 69
limitations of adaptive statistical
    techniques, 69–71
methodologies for allocating alpha,
    60–62
    Bonferroni correction, 60–61
    Holm correction, 61
    other methods, 61–62
misconception about p values, 58–59
Monte Carlo simulation, 72
nominal p values, 57
noninferiority studies, 88
null hypothesis, 70
outcome dependent randomization,
    83
outcome values, 73
patient participation, duration of, 76
placebo, 59, 84
Pocock's method, 63
posterior distribution, 71
primary endpoint, 80, 87
prior distribution, 71
program failure, 91

random highs (group sequential
    designs), 90
recursive techniques, 67
repeated significance tests, 63
self-designing studies, 68
simulations and modeling, 72–73
statistical analysis plan, 62
statistically significant results, 57
stopping boundaries, 63
Student-Newman-Keuls test, 61
treatment effect, estimates of, 85
trial simulations, 92
Tukey's test, 61
Type I error inflation, 55
unblinded analysis, 65
uncertainty, modeled sources of, 91
variability data, 60
variance spending, 66
virtual experiments, 72
STER, *see* Strict TER
Strict TER (STER), 132, 133
Student-Newman-Keuls (SNK) test, 61
Study, *see also* Trial
    adequate and well-controlled
      studies, 75
    changes, types of, 10
    conditions for termination, 9
    confirmatory, 18
    databases, 35
    dose selection, 81
    faulty design, 163
    integrity, 29
    internal pilot, 114
    interventional, 44
    learning, 18
    length, 96
    non-adaptive, 8
    noninferiority, 88
    non-pivotal, 27
    observational, 44
    oncology, 132, 136, 140
    pharmacokinetic, change in dosage,
      7
    Phase I
      alpha preservation, 140
      classic designs, 131
      continual reassessment method,
        134
      data collection, 4

dose escalation, 124, 137
dosing, 11
individual sequential designs, 145
learning trials, 130
multiple ascending dose study, 125
oncology studies, 132
purpose, 2
risk of, 3, 10, 117
stochastic approximation method,
    138
Phase II
    adaptive changes in dosing for,
        130
    designed as hypothesis testing
        studies, 3
    heterogeneity of, 2
    location scale, 152
Phase III
    confirm type of trial, 13
    location scale, 152
    Provenge, 21
    safety and efficacy establishment
        using, 2
Phase IV, 2
pivotal, dose adaptation in, 140–141
placebo-controlled, 98
prospective, 44
retrospective, 44
self-designing, 9, 68
termination, 39, 78–80, *see also*
    Interim analysis and adaptive
    termination of study and study
    arms
titration, 127
traditional, 37
underpowered, 111
validity of, 1
Study design and decision rules,
        adaptive changes in, 149–153
    Bauer method, 150, 151
    decision rules, 149
    endpoints and hypothesis, changing
        of, 150–151
        blinded data, 150
        unblinded data, 150–151
    flexible designs, 149–150
    follow-up period, changes to, 149

Herceptin, 152
overview, 149
per patient population, definition of,
    151
Phase III studies, 152
placebo effect, 150
reactive clinical trial design, 150
reverse multiplicity, 152
statistical analysis plan, 151
test statistic or analysis, changes to,
    151–152
    blinded data, 151
    unblinded data, 151–152
Type I error, 149
variance spending approach, 150
Survivor bias, 165
Systematic bias, 23, 24

T

Tables, listings, and graphs (TLGs), 13
Tachyphylaxis, 129, 168
Tenecteplase (tPA), 165
TER, *see* Traditional escalation rule
Test
    exact, 171
    Holm *t*, 61
    parametric, 51
    permutation, 171
    randomization, 171
    repeated significance, 63
    statistical, types of, 51, 52, *see also*
        Statistics
    Student-Newman-Keuls, 61
    Tukey's, 61
    variable, 47
    z-, 50
Therapeutic ratio, 119
Therapeutic–response curve, 17, 18
Time-to-event continual reassessment
        method (TITE-CRM), 136
TITE-CRM, *see* Time-to-event continual
        reassessment method
Titrated dosing, 124
TLGs, *see* Tables, listings, and graphs
tPA, *see* Tenecteplase
Traditional escalation rule (TER), 132

Trial, *see also* Study
  analysis, 17
  assignment, 17
  conduct, *see* Seamless designs and
      adaptive clinical trial conduct
  confirming, 16, 17
  descriptive, 16
  design, 66
  endpoint, 168
  goals, 25
  hypothesis-confirming, 27
  integrity, 170
  learning phase, 16
  observation, 17
  reasons for stopping, 145
  simulations, 91, 92
  types, 13
Tukey's test, 61
Type I error
  avoided, 23
  control, 6, 20, 76
  frequentist rubric, 24
  inflation, 55, 89, 171
  interim analysis and, 6
  preserved, 66
  probability of, 56
  rate, 84
  risk, 22, 61
  statistical calculations of, 161
Type II error
  avoided, 23
  rate, inflation of, 89
  reduced levels, 24
  treatment effect and, 90
  underpowered studies and, 111

U

Unblinded analyses, 65
Unblinded data, 113, 150–151
U.S. Food and Drug Administration
    (FDA), 2, 56
  adaptive design protocols, 159
  alpha preservation, 27
  Bayesian statistics, 30
  drug approval, replication
      requirement, 28

  flexible designs, 28
  guidance document on adaptive
      studies, 20
  endpoints, 20
  patient evaluations, 20
  sample size, 20
  study eligibility criteria, 20
  treatment regimens, 20
  non-pivotal studies, 27
  nuisance parameters, 27
  regulatory guidance, 30–36
    early and middle period of drug
        development, 31
    evaluating and reporting
        completed study, 34–36
    late stages of drug development,
        31–32
    special protocol assessments,
        32–33
    study blinding and information
        sharing, 33–34
  special protocol assessments, 28
  study integrity, 29
U.S. Food and Drug Administration,
    stance on adaptive techniques,
    73–93
  adaptive study designs whose
      properties are less well
      understood, 81–88
  dose selection studies, 81–83
  endpoint selection, 86–87
  interim effect size estimates,
      84–85
  multiple-study design features in
      single study, 87–88
  noninferiority studies, 88
  patient population, 85–86
  relative treatment group
      responses, 83–84
  statistical considerations for less
      well-understood adaptive
      design methods, 89–93
  clinical trial simulation, 91–92
  increased Type II error rate, 90–91
  prospective statistical analysis
      plan, 92–93
  statistical bias, 90

study-wide Type I error rate,
  89–90
valid approaches to implementation,
  74–81
  adaptations in data analysis plan,
    80–81
  blinded interim analysis of
    aggregate data, 75–76
  early study termination, 78–80
  outcome unrelated to efficacy,
    76–78
  study eligibility criteria, 74–75

V

Variance spending, 66, 113, 150
Virtual experiments, 72

W

Water-soluble drugs, 121

Z

z-test, 50

Milton Keynes UK
Ingram Content Group UK Ltd.
UKHW040056071024
449327UK00019B/594

9 780367 382476